THE
PRESCRIPTION-
TO-PRISON PIPELINE

THE PRESCRIPTION- TO-PRISON

Duke University Press *Durham and London* 2023

PIPELINE

THE MEDICALIZATION

AND CRIMINALIZATION OF PAIN

Michelle Smirnova

Printed and bound by CPI Group (UK) Ltd, Croydon, CR0 4YY
Project Editor: Liz Smith
Designed by Courtney Leigh Richardson
Typeset in Portrait and Trade Gothic by Westchester Publishing Services

Library of Congress Cataloging-in-Publication Data
Names: Smirnova, Michelle, [date] author.
Title: The prescription-to-prison pipeline : the medicalization and criminalization
of pain / Michelle Smirnova.
Description: Durham : Duke University Press, 2023. | Includes bibliographical references
and index.
Identifiers: LCCN 2022041333 (print)
LCCN 2022041334 (ebook)
ISBN 9781478019695 (paperback)
ISBN 9781478017066 (hardcover)
ISBN 9781478024330 (ebook)
Subjects: LCSH: Opioid abuse—Social aspects—United States. | Medication abuse—Social
aspects—United States. | Drug abuse—Government policy—United States. | Discrimination in
law enforcement—United States. | Discrimination in criminal justice administration—United
States. | BISAC: SOCIAL SCIENCE / Sociology / General | SOCIAL SCIENCE / Anthropology /
Cultural & Social
Classification: LCC HV5825 .S56 2023 (print) | LCC HV5825 (ebook) |
DDC 362.29/30973—dc23/eng/20221214
LC record available at https://lccn.loc.gov/2022041333
LC ebook record available at https://lccn.loc.gov/2022041334

Cover art: Pills. © Peter Dazeley. Courtesy Getty Images and the artist.

CONTENTS

ACKNOWLEDGMENTS

This book project began with Jennifer Owens. As two newly minted assistant professors, Jena and I sat next to each other on the orientation bus on our first day employed at the University of Missouri–Kansas City. We chatted about our respective moves from Washington, DC, and St. Louis, Missouri; about the pleasant surprise of housing costs and walkable commutes to school. Then we asked each other about what we were up to: our research. Jena's dissertation had focused on methamphetamine use and production among women. I had been working on a broad assortment of projects, ranging from studies of political humor as resistance to the medicalization of youth. She asked me what I meant by medicalization, as she was curious about this novel concept. She asked if it included prescription drugs. Many of the women she had interviewed had told her she should be paying attention to prescription drugs rather than illicit ones—they were the real problem these days. We chatted about this—I offered some theories why that might be the case—but then we changed the subject to discuss more important things, such as where to get good Korean food in Kansas City.

Later that year, Jena walked into my office and asked whether I'd be interested in working on a project with her. She wanted to go into prisons and ask women about prescription drugs. She knew that I was a trained methodologist, given both my graduate preparation and my two years of working in the qualitative research center at the United States Census Bureau, so she thought I could help design the surveys and interview instruments as well as collect the data. I was interested. We drafted several grants and began the long Institutional Review Board (IRB) process for approval. Over the next three years, we applied for five grants, interviewed eighty incarcerated people, surveyed over five hundred individuals, and made many, many long car trips together. During these trips, we processed our interviews, discussed politics and books, and questioned how *America's Funniest Home Videos* was still in existence after the advent of YouTube and TikTok. Jena has since left higher education, but I cannot imagine how I would have set off on this project without her. She is one of the most detail-oriented research partners, and she taught me how to be a more attentive researcher and scholar.

Jena and I were part of a UM system program called the Faculty Scholars, through which we went on retreats to develop our research, apply for grants, and learn new teaching techniques. It was on this retreat that I met other faculty whom I could laugh and commiserate with, including Amanda Grimes, Debra Leiter, Jamie Hunt, David Thurmaier, Jason Martin, Sarah Marie Martin, and Lori Sexton. I am grateful to the UM system for providing this program, which helped connect me with other new professors who ultimately became part of my support (read: survival) network in my early years as an assistant professor. The university was not equally supportive of all of us, and, in witnessing those inequities, I think about how we might change structures and cultures to change that every day.

Lori Sexton is the type of colleague and friend who will convince you that there is brilliance and humor on even the greyest days. Our regular coffee-shop dates have helped me process my research, teaching, and life in invaluable ways. Lori read an early version of this manuscript and offered thoughtful feedback. Given her extensive research in prisons and focus on restorative justice, she helped frame this book in important ways.

Jenny Huberman managed to read the entire first draft of this book and provide comments in less than a week's time. Jenny has been my across-the-hall mentor and one of my closest friends since I started at UMKC. Jenny and Jeff welcomed me into their home and family from the moment I arrived in Kansas City and gave me the first sense of community. Not only has Jenny helped me process this research at its many stages of development, but she is also responsible for making Kansas City feel like home.

Others at UMKC who helped the book come to be include Debbie Smith, the chair of the sociology department during these six years. She was supportive of the project from the beginning and wrote in support of me for several grants and awards related to the project. The Women's and Sexualities Studies Department provided two crucial early grants to start this research and the Funding for Excellence Grants secured us enough funding to bring this project to fruition. Makini King and Sandy Rodriguez shaped my thinking at the later stages of this work—when I was already revising the manuscript—but I am immensely grateful for their friendship and intellectual guidance.

To Gisela Fosado, Ale Mejía, and the entire Duke editorial, production, and marketing teams: this book would not be here were it not for your tireless labor. Gisela, in particular, saw value in my project from its inception, fought for its publication, and was my biggest advocate and supporter throughout the process. Ale made the process clear, seamless, and expedient and was always a pleasure to work with. The two of them were also responsible for identifying and working with the two anonymous reviewers of this manuscript, who provided invaluable feedback. Each of the reviewers, along with Gisela, seemed truly invested in growing this book into its best possible form. I am incredibly grateful for their meticulous and thoughtful readings and their copious constructive and transformative commentary. I know this labor is uncompensated and often thankless, but I can truly say that this book would not be what it is without you, so I am most appreciative that I was able to benefit from all your labor and investment in this project.

While friends and mentors from graduate school did not all read this book, it often felt like they were sitting in the room as I typed, reminding me to be thoughtful and careful with my analyses and interpretations. Aleia Clark was one of my closest graduate school comrades. I pegged her as my friend on the first day of the program and am grateful she didn't completely rebuke me, as I'm not sure I would have survived without her. I called Aleia many times while I worked on this book, and as always, she was able to see clearly though the haze, helping me make important theoretical connections and practical decisions. Melissa Milkie has been a mentor and a close friend for the past fifteen years. Everyone should find their "Melissa" (though it's unlikely the knockoff version will be as good as the original). She is notorious among graduate students (and professors and friends) as being an unwavering source of support and motivation. I don't think I could have made it through graduate school or completed this book without her support. Melissa encouraged me to get involved with the Sociologists for Women in Society, and those conferences have felt like a retreat from this world—where we biked, hiked, and danced our way through mountains, sessions, and research projects.

People often say that once you learn sociology, it is difficult to "unsee" it. I feel the same way about Patricia Hill Collins, fondly known as "PHC," and her groundbreaking work on intersectionality and the matrix of domination. She has shaped my worldview and research in ways that become increasingly apparent over the years. I am grateful for her patience and humor as a professor and a mentor. Laura Mamo, Emily Mann, Carolina Martin, Tony Hatch, and Valerie Chepp are other inspiring sociologists who shaped my thinking during graduate school and shaped this book. Laura Mamo first introduced me to medical sociology and science and technology studies, and it's hard to imagine this book without those classes I took early in graduate school. Emily Mann read an early version of one paper that served as the backbone for this project and provided attentive feedback as well as generously connecting me to other scholars doing similar work. Carolina Martin was a buoy through graduate school as well as the years that followed. Valerie Chepp showed me how it was possible to juggle more than I thought was possible. Tony Hatch read an early chapter of the book and helped identify central mechanisms and concerns of the prescription-to-prison pipeline.

In addition to my academic community, there are many others in my life who shaped this book. My friends in DC: Natalie, Lena, Sara, Jimmy, Jon, Emmy—I am eternally grateful for your friendship, love, and inspiration to fight for a more just and equitable world. Julia and Aliza, while we haven't lived nearby since college, I'm so energized each time we visit or get off the phone. Although I didn't know anyone in Kansas City prior to starting my position at UMKC, CDV, an important connector in our lives, connected me to Quinton—a fellow Wash U alum who also lived in KC. We met on a job visit and immediately hit it off. Q is one of the wittiest, smartest, and most welcoming people out there, and he introduced us to half the people we know in KC today. Debates about drug policy, homelessness, and medicalization were common dinner table conversation with Meghan, Jeff, Caety, Matt, Katherine, and Q, as were they around the fire pit with Matthew, Louisa, Becca, and Jordan. Each of you shaped my thinking in important ways. To Mary, Kevin, Jennifer, Ryan, Chris, Darin, and Maggie, thanks for bringing hilarity and joy to our lives. To all of our Kansas City family, thank you for welcoming us with open arms and making this city feel like home.

Lauren and Jess, my two longest friends and my chosen sisters, I am forever grateful to have you as family and to have you there to lift me up when I need it the most. You remind me to celebrate my victories and are always there to assist in that endeavor. You both challenge and inspire me and I always look forward to being able to process the world with you.

Thank you to my mom, who is similarly there to shower me with love and support and who has served as a role model of how one might persevere through all the challenges of life—emigrating to a new country as a refugee, learning to speak a new language, and building a new community and career. As she always reminds me, find something that you love and fight for it.

AJ, you are that something. I'm so grateful for you now and always. You are brilliant, kind, and more humble than anyone else I know. You inspire, support, and love me in a way that makes me aspire to be my best self. You and Zev keep me grounded and full of love. I love the way you see and engage with the world, and I always appreciate your thoughtful reflections and feedback. I just wish you'd read Marx already.

Finally, I'd like to extend my gratitude and appreciation to the individuals who participated in the surveys and interviews. Thank you for trusting me with your stories and for offering your candid insights and reflections. Without you, this book would not exist. I hope this book does justice to your lives and that it effects positive changes that you experience firsthand.

INTRODUCTION

QUICK FIXES TO ENDURING PROBLEMS

I met Lyndsey when she was forty-five years old. A petite blonde woman with bright blue eyes, she sat across a table from me, taking up half of an aluminum metal chair. For the duration of our conversation, she sat folded in upon herself, her hands clasped around her crossed legs, gently rubbing one thumb over the other. She responded to most questions with an affirmative "yes ma'am" while looking me in the eyes, or "no, ma'am," looking down. We sat in an undecorated office that looked like it could have been anywhere in corporate America. But its door was much heavier and it did not lock, unlike the prison cell down the hall where Lyndsey had spent the last three years serving a sentence for operating a motor vehicle while under the influence of pharmaceutical drugs that had not been prescribed to her.

While her life was not always easy, no one expected Lyndsey to end up in prison. Lyndsey developed leukemia at a young age and spent a lot of time in the care of doctors. Despite this harrowing, potentially fatal diagnosis, symptoms of her illness were slow to develop, especially in her youth. While she tried to keep an optimistic outlook—which was evident as she described her aspirations for college and travel upon completion of her sentence—her life always felt precarious. It was unclear how long she would have or which milestones she would live to see. Lyndsey dreamed of a big wedding, followed by a big family, attending college to become a teacher—then therapist, then social worker.

Despite these ambitions, she knew better than to live for the future when the present was perpetually uncertain. Lyndsey grew up poor in a household where she was regularly abused both physically and sexually. Her father terrorized her mother and siblings, often pitting them against each other so that the fear permeated the house even in his absence. Two of her sisters were removed by Child Protective Services, though for reasons unknown to Lyndsey, she and her other siblings remained within her father's custody. Guilt, fear, and anger were emotions that Lyndsey became familiar with at an early age.

As a result of this upbringing, Lyndsey was elated when she found out she was pregnant at seventeen years old. She had always dreamed about starting a family of her own, and she and her boyfriend had decided to get married and raise their child. The baby meant she could escape her father, the abuse, and her diagnosis of leukemia. She loved being pregnant—with a child and with dreams of a hopeful future. But then, at eight months pregnant, Lyndsey's red blood cell count dropped to worrisome levels. The doctors performed an emergency cesarean section in order to save her child. The baby survived the delivery, but his lungs were underdeveloped. He was transferred to the NICU, where he spent several months, but his lungs continued to collapse even with the additional support. At three months old, Lyndsey's baby developed pneumonia and died.

Lyndsey was devastated. She had lost her son. The marriage soon fell apart as well. Everything began to unravel again. While she had had a difficult childhood and battle with leukemia, her pregnancy and potential marriage had given her hope for a better life. When her baby died, she was shattered.

In the wake of her baby's birth, Lyndsey was prescribed Xanax to manage her anxiety, depression, and persistent panic attacks. She was also prescribed Vicodin to moderate the pain from her C-section. Although she had been prescribed pain medication many times before for surgeries and chronic pain related to her leukemia, this time, she had trouble coming off them. She continued to experience both physical and psychological pain, and she found that the Vicodin helped provide her with energy, which helped her hold down a job and support herself. The prescriptions were keeping her going.

But after some time, seemingly out of nowhere, her doctors stopped refilling the scripts. Lyndsey didn't know what to do; the withdrawal was torture, and without the medications, she couldn't motivate herself to get out of bed. One friend connected her with someone to sell her Xanax to help manage withdrawal symptoms. Another suggested she try methamphetamine instead of the Vicodin to give her energy. Medicating herself with these cobbled prescriptions and substances, Lyndsey was able to hold down her job, support and care for her family, and spend time with friends. Things were looking up. But then she was pulled over and her car was searched. They found a pill bottle that didn't have her name on it. Arrested and sentenced to five years in prison, Lyndsey told me her story.

Seven in ten adults in the United States take a prescription drug on a daily basis.[1] One in five takes at least one prescribed psychotropic drug, and one in three has been prescribed an opioid painkiller.[2] Psychotropics are substances that change brain chemistry and affect the functioning of the central nervous system. They include a broad range of prescription drugs including tranquilizers that are used to manage anxiety and panic disorders (e.g., benzodiazepines, Xanax), stimulants used to amplify perception (e.g., Adderall), and sedatives or hypnotics used to treat insomnia (e.g., Ambien). They are prescribed with increasing frequency to anyone exhibiting psychiatric distress (as defined by health professionals) and are increasingly likely to be prescribed by primary care doctors rather than psychiatrists.

Opioid pain killers are prescription medications that have the ability to quell pain. The morphine molecule—the primary chemical compound in opium—is designed to overwhelm our bodies' mu-opioid receptors, which produce a pleasurable sensation similar to that which is produced when natural endorphins are released in the body. As psychotropics are increasingly used as a cure-all for psychiatric distress, opioids are seen as a panacea for treating physical pain.

The ubiquity and normalization of prescription drug consumption have contributed to what anthropologist Joseph Dumit has termed "drugs for life."[3] Instead of being used to treat visible symptoms or prevent death, pharmaceuticals are being used to increase and augment quality of life. The power of medicine and drugs has expanded with the increased medicalization of the social world, whereby previously nonmedical experiences, such as sadness or addiction, come to be defined as medical problems, illnesses, or disorders. In doing so, the medical model locates problems in the bodies of individuals rather than social contexts, relegating responsibility (and blame) to those individuals rather than to policies, laws, or social inequalities.[4]

This process is what sociologists often refer to as "medicalization"—the process by which nonmedical problems are transformed into biological issues to be treated with medical intervention. Just as many endemic social problems are being medicalized and treated with *medical* substances, *nonmedical* substance use is being increasingly criminalized and treated with incarceration or other forms of institutionalization.

In the last forty years, the number of people incarcerated on drug charges has risen tenfold—from 40,900 in 1980 to 452,900 in 2017[5]—due to sentencing policies that were developed as part of what is often termed the "War on Drugs." Today, half a million people are behind bars on any given night for a drug law violation—ten times the number in 1980.[6] Specifically, 56 percent of women and 47 percent of men in federal prisons are serving time for drug-related offenses.[7] Fifty-eight percent of those in juvenile correctional facilities are also there because of drug-related charges.[8] Even those who do not serve time in jail or prison for a drug conviction suffer potential social, economic, and political consequences for their substance use in many states, including the loss of child custody, employment, student aid, public housing, public assistance, and the right to vote. Fifty-eight percent of federal prisoners and 47 percent of state prisoners are parents.[9] As a consequence, millions of children in the United States grow up without a parent. The vast majority of those parents (two-thirds) are incarcerated for nonviolent offenses, such as drug law violations.[10]

Drug use is often treated as deviant behavior that occurs outside of mainstream society, despite the fact that pharmaceuticals are prescribed by doctors at historic rates and that a significant proportion of people (one in five in the United States) have used an illicit substance in the past year.[11] In 2018, almost seventeen million people in the United States had used a prescription psychotherapeutic drug without the oversight of a doctor in the past year, which constitutes illegal use.[12] According to the Controlled Substances Act, prescription drugs are classified as a controlled substance; therefore, if used "in a manner or amount inconsistent with the legitimate medical use," this use of prescription drugs is considered "drug abuse" and is punishable by law.[13]

The use of prescription drugs without a doctor's supervision is considered to be *nonmedical*. The qualifier "nonmedical" denotes the fact that these substances are used without the direct oversight of a doctor as is assumed with *medical* prescription drug use.[14] Some nonmedical use involves substances that were prescribed by a doctor but are used in greater quantities than prescribed or consumed in a different mode than prescribed (i.e., crushed and snorted or injected intravenously to produce a more potent and immediate effect). Other times, nonmedical use refers to the fact that the pills were obtained from sources other than a doctor, including family members or acquaintances.

The term *nonmedical use* is used in this book rather than *abuse* given that *abuse* implies harm, an assumption that is used by the medical and legal establishments to justify coercive treatment or punishment. While substance use under a doctor's supervision is considered to be beneficial at best and harmless at worst, independent substance use is exclusively constructed as harmful, even when the specific modality, quantity, or purpose of use is identical to that occurring under a doctor's supervision, as was mostly the case with Lyndsey and others interviewed for this book. The power of medical and carceral systems lies in their ability to define and thereby control populations. This occurs through individual actors, such as doctors or judges, but also through institutionalized classificatory systems, such as the *Diagnostic and Statistical Manual of Mental Disorders* (DSM), which is used by psychiatrists to diagnose and treat psychiatric disorders.

In this book, I argue that medicalization and criminalization work together to intensify harm among already marginalized individuals like Lyndsey. This intensification occurs in a number of ways. It begins with the classification of certain behaviors as harms that warrant surveillance and intervention. In so doing, we lose the opportunity to understand the motivation or purpose of a behavior as it has been simplistically reduced to a disease or a crime. We listen to representatives of medical and legal institutions diagnose and pass judgment without entertaining the possibility that the patient or defendant has a greater perspective on the context and on their embodied experience. Once a person is labeled an "addict" or a "criminal," their agency and trustworthiness diminish. The medicalization and criminalization of a behavior justify medical and legal intervention, control, and punishment, all of which can be accomplished under the guise of benevolence, of helping or "treating" individuals. Yet the individual is rarely listened to or treated as a collaborator in their own care.

The second way that medicalization and criminalization can produce more harm is through techniques that produce the very problems they allege to treat. A great example of this is overdose. While in theory, medical and legal systems aim to *prevent* or *treat* overdose, their practices often *produce* overdose as well. The criminalization of nonmedical substance use forces substances underground, where it can be difficult to account for potency or purity of what one ingests and which forces individuals into secrecy, whereby they use alone or under conditions of duress. Each of these factors increases the likelihood of overdose. People who have been incarcerated are more likely to overdose as they experience forcible withdrawal while in prison and have diminished tolerance upon release. With few support systems in place to assist them back into a world where they experience barriers to housing, employment, and social support, many return to managing problems through medications that their bodies are no longer prepared to handle. This can also result in overdose. In fact, one study finds that in the first two weeks after being released, former prisoners were forty times more likely to die of an opioid overdose than the general population. Even after a year, overdose rates remained between ten and eighteen times higher among the formerly incarcerated than among the general population.[15] These data alone challenge the notion that criminalizing substance use reduces overdose incidence. Instead, it may increase it.

Third, the medicalization and criminalization of "addiction" (established as a primary risk factor for overdose) further exacerbate harm as they extend punishment across the expansive industry of drug courts, rehabilitation programs, and prisons. Under the guise of "therapeutic jurisprudence," the legal system has joined forces with health-care providers to treat individuals deemed "at risk" of overdose. As a result, one's risk factors for addiction—substance use, unemployment, failure to pay a bill—become signs of medical and criminal risk. This warrants simultaneous medical and legal intervention to protect the individual from harm, despite the fact that the programs themselves produce greater harm by convincing individuals that they are "irresponsible addicts," forcibly removing them from their families and communities, and permanently marking both their medical and legal records, thus thwarting access to employment, housing, and education, all of which are directly correlated with positive health outcomes.

Finally, the dominant paradigm in the United States of punitive approach to substance use only intensifies all the harms outlined above. Previous scholarship has challenged the notion that drug courts and rehabilitation programs offer more humane alternatives to incarceration.[16] In fact, they extend and exacerbate punishment, as people who participate in drug courts and mandatory rehabilitation programs often serve longer prison sentences than those who do not and are subject to psychological punishment in addition to isolation and traditional penal practices.[17] Perpetual surveillance can create a self-fulfilling prophecy. Prior to incarceration, as part of mandatory rehabilitation programs, or after release, as part of probation and parole requirements, individuals are subject to regular state surveillance. This can intensify anxiety and stress as the looming threat of reincarceration accompanies otherwise mundane experiences such as getting stuck in traffic on one's way home from work in time for a court-mandated curfew. The incarcerated also bear the cost of their incarceration, as individuals must pay for GPS ankle monitors, drug and alcohol monitoring bracelets, and other biometric and surveillance technologies. The financial, social, and psychological effects of isolation are further intensified by new techniques of rehabilitative punishment that convinces individuals that they are fundamentally flawed and in need of psychological transformation. As a consequence, punishment is exacerbated not only in terms of breadth, via extended prison sentences and state surveillance, but also in terms of depth, as they must internalize the punishment process as panoptic prisoner-patients.[18]

This book builds upon this scholarship by foregrounding the narratives of eighty incarcerated individuals who experienced the effects of having their lives both medicalized and criminalized. Bearing witness to their stories, the book demonstrates how medical and legal systems often work in ways that intensify—rather than ameliorate—endemic social problems. In doing so, they both produce and exacerbate inequalities along the lines of race, class, and gender.

This is not to put blame on the shoulders of medical or legal professionals, as many people who go into these fields do so with the intention of helping rather than hurting. The problem is that social issues such as those covered in this book—including child abuse; poverty; unemployment; interpersonal violence; inequities in education, health care, or wages; racism in policing and incarceration; and lack of affordable childcare or support for new mothers—should be attended to through structural rather than individual-level solutions. In the United States, such issues are often presented as individual-level problems and thereby treated with individual-level solutions. And yet individual-level solutions, such as medication, treatment, or incarceration, often only make matters worse.

In this book, I trace how nonmedical prescription drug use may be seen as the result of the intersection of three social processes: (1) structural inequalities in the US system that simultaneously produce unequal levels of pain and unequal access to health care, (2) the medicalization and pharmaceuticalization of pain, and (3) an ongoing War on Drugs that produces and maintains axes of inequality along the lines of race, class, and gender through the criminalization of substance use in addition to inequitable policing and incarcerating practices. Using the narratives of incarcerated persons who used prescription drugs nonmedically, I illustrate how they did (and do) so in order to cope with an unequal system, but also to resist institutions that classify, diagnose, treat, and punish.

The Power of Contradictions

Regulation of prescription drug use in the United States involves a number of contradictions, which effectively challenge fundamental assumptions that are used to justify legislation. For example, many licit prescription drugs are almost identical in chemical construction to other substances classified as *illicit* (e.g., opioids versus opium, amphetamines versus methamphetamines). Prescription drug use is deemed legal and safe when used in certain contexts, but illegal in others: an individual can use a substance legally if it is prescribed by a doctor, but if they continue to use that drug or obtain it from a source other than a doctor, it is illegal and punishable by law. "Off-label" prescribing, where doctors prescribe a drug for a condition other than the one approved by the US Food and Drug Administration, is legal and common. And yet, nonmedical prescription drug use among nonlicensed persons is criminalized. The same decade that the World Health Organization (WHO) declared "freedom from pain" as a universal human right,[19] warranting liberal prescription of pain medication, the United States declared its War on Drugs, thereby criminalizing all other substance use. A drug is considered to be *abused* if one intends to use it for pleasure; however, opioids and other pharmaceutical drugs are designed specifically to activate endorphins or block the reuptake of serotonin—mechanisms to promote the biological production of pleasure. The criminalization of substance use has historically been a tool for locking up people of color. However, as more white people are being incarcerated, we have witnessed a "therapeutic turn" from punishment to treatment of substance use, illustrating how colorblind legislation continues to be implemented in racially unjust ways.

These contradictions raise important questions. If the boundaries between pleasure and productivity, use and abuse, and licit and illicit substances are much more amorphous than we are led to believe, how are we to police or legislate them? How does the shift from measurable harm to perceived risk cause disadvantaged "at risk" groups to come under greater scrutiny, surveillance, and punishment for the same actions committed by "nonrisky" groups? How do these contradictions produce unequal outcomes for individuals using prescription drugs?

These contradictions might also be perceived to be intentional as they position institutions and authorities to be the arbiters of truth and the associated consequences. People in power get to answer these questions and codify them in new laws, policies, and practices, while those directly impacted by these decisions are rarely consulted in serious or meaningful ways.

This book expands beyond the well-worn narrative of the opioid or overdose crisis by encouraging policy makers, politicians, and the voters who elect them to see the crisis as a social—rather than biological or pharmaceutical—problem. The term *opioid epidemic* implies that (1) we are dealing with a new problem that is caused exclusively by opioids, and (2) opioids are exclusively harmful. Yet opioids are not new. Opium, as derived from opium poppies, has been used to both quell pain and produce joy for millennia.[20] Morphine was first synthesized from opium in 1805 and was subsequently prescribed for everything ranging from pain to respiratory illness to cough to diarrhea. While more limited in application, opiates continue to be considered beneficial and are widely encouraged in medical settings. Further, most negative outcomes associated with opioids are the product of polydrug use rather than opioids in isolation. Framing the situation as an opioid crisis is reductive, and it also misdirects our attention to the "simple" issues of purity and potency and distracts "from the social, political, and economic conditions that make overdose deaths more likely in some situations and less likely in others."[21]

In other words, the language of "epidemics" obscures endemic social conditions that produce harm. If opiates or other substances were the exclusive—or even primary—cause of these harms, eliminating them would be the solution. And yet, we see how opiates and other prescription drugs are not outlawed, how they continue to be prescribed by doctors, and how those in pain benefit from their use. We also find that the outlawing of opiates—or other substances—does not reduce poverty, incarceration, unemployment, or overdose. In fact, policing, legislating, and punishing substance use only *increases* these harms. The true causes of these harms—endemic structural poverty, racism, genderism, and sexism—are rendered *invisible* by the language of opioid and overdose crises. Those who navigate what sociologist Celeste Watkins-Hayes terms "injuries of inequality" on a daily basis are ignored until they end up in hospitals, rehab centers, prison, or graves.[22] Only then do they receive interventions or support—or, at least, they make a news headline as a statistic. Further, much of the media coverage of the "opioid epidemic" specifically centers rural white and middle-class communities, deflecting attention from urban communities of color that have been subject to policing, incarceration, and overdose for decades with little media attention, empathy, or push for meaningful policy reform.[23] Historically, drug policy has done more to harm than to protect communities of color in the United States.[24]

The language of epidemics and crises "misrepresent[s] the duration and scale of the situation," given that the issues raised are in fact *ordinary* rather than *extraordinary* features of US society.[25] To borrow the language of cultural theorist Lauren Berlant, many of these individuals had long been enduring a "slow death" prior to the statistical crisis of an overdose or arrest. The term *slow death* refers to "the destruction of bodies by capitalism in spaces of production and in the rest of life," such as the injuries, stress, and traumas produced by long hours, insufficient wages, and precarious conditions of capitalist work and life that often disproportionately impact "vulnerable populations, which include people of color and the aged, but more broadly, too, the economically crunched."[26] For such groups, slow death is the result of a society defined by inequality and the objectification of one's labor and body. Rather than an aberration or "epidemic" caused by a substance, such exploitation and its health consequences are a "defining condition of their experience and historical existence."[27] Treating such structural inequality as a novel event is a strategy for mitigating guilt or shame by a society that is complicit in that harm by not engaging in the "heroic agency a crisis seems already to have called for."[28]

The issues bundled in the "opioid epidemic" are not limited to overdose and death but also include incarceration, unemployment, chronic pain, depression, anxiety, trauma, abuse, and violence. These are not the product of a disease, disaster, or isolated injury, they are a product of structural inequities. As science historian Nancy Campbell argues, they reflect a "human-made disaster exacerbated by denial and disavowal of responsibility by those who structured and maintained distinctions between legal and illegal drugs, 'patients' and 'addicts,' and physiological and existential pain."[29] However, these issues are also the responsibility of those who participate in and uphold a society that fails to provide individuals who suffer from these issues with dignity or provide them with appropriate care.

We are all implicated in this system of inequality and its casualties. This is not to say that it is everyone's responsibility and, therefore, effectively no one's. Quite the opposite. Those of us with greater privilege and power—by virtue of our skin color, gender, wealth, occupation, or influence over institutional policy and action—are more culpable and therefore must engage in more extensive undoing. But we all perpetuate such inequalities in some ways at ideological or institutional levels, and therefore it is a collective project. Above all else, constructing these issues as individual rather than collective or structural is at the heart of the problem. This is often accomplished through the medical and legal institutions of our society and is why they are the focus of this book.

At Risk of Social Control: Medicalization of Structural Inequalities

Philosopher Michel Foucault argued that contemporary power—what he terms "biopower"—is productive rather than repressive.[30] It produces bodies, identities, and new ways of processing the world. It establishes new standards, new ways of knowing about human life, and new aspirational goals. It comes to determine what is a (good) life, and what is not. Biopower is enacted via modern state institutions that collect and legislate upon population-level data, but it is also internalized by individuals who come to understand themselves through biopolitical discourse. In so doing, it has subsumed the structure-agency balance of power, whereby individuals perceive themselves to be thinking and acting independently and distinctively. The aim of biopolitical power is to increase productivity of the body and society in tandem, quantified by such epidemiological population measures as birth, morbidity, and mortality rates as well as economic measures of gross domestic product (GDP) and employment rates.[31]

This quest for productivity is facilitated by the medicalization process that supports or thwarts behaviors, bodies, and ideas based on their alignment with contemporary notions of productivity. The term *medicalization* was first used in the 1970s by sociologist Irving K. Zola and medical philosopher Ivan Illich to describe how previously nonmedical experiences, such as sadness or addiction, came to be defined as medical problems, illnesses, or disorders.[32] From their perspective, health care had become a "sick-making enterprise" in which doctors and medicine are responsible for *producing* rather than *curing* diseases.[33] As a result, many problems become medical rather than social, political, or financial. Individuals are transformed from citizens and community members into lifelong patients dependent upon the services of doctors, medicine, and health care. Medicine is not merely a source of treatment, but it is a source of identity. This is made particularly possible through prescription drugs.

Prescription drugs are a medical technology, not unlike the giant machines hooked up to patients in hospital beds.[34] These small pills have reconstituted health care and medicine both within and outside the clinical setting. People take pills with their morning coffee or before brushing their teeth at night. They occupy our most intimate spaces—bedside tables, purses, desks drawers at work. They are ubiquitous to contemporary US life. Yet, while they require self-administration, self-diagnosis and self-treatment remain prohibited. They require the internalization of medical discourse and the medical gaze, whereby an individual must surveil and treat their body and brain according to how health professionals deem fit.[35] Yet this surveillance of body and mind and associated medication or treatment are often experienced as a personal decision or ambition, as medical treatment becomes a type of identity work. This is particularly true with pharmaceutical drugs.

Pharmaceuticalization refers to the redefinition and reconstruction of social or structural problems as having a pharmaceutical solution,[36] such as the prescription of antianxiety medication to soldiers returning from war or restless children being prescribed Ritalin to help them sit still in school. Pharmaceuticalization has been made possible by the rise of autonomous consumer-patients,[37] the availability of more products over the counter without a doctor's oversight,[38] the use of certain prescription drugs for "enhancement" purposes (e.g., Viagra),[39] and the increasing marketing influence of pharmaceutical companies, amid lighter media regulation.[40]

Pharmaceutical drugs are used more widely in the contemporary United States than in any other geographic region or historical period.[41] This is also the result of the ever-expanding realm of conditions and experiences that have become pharmaceuticalized. By constructing social problems as biological ones, pharmaceutical companies, scientists, doctors, and legislators offer pharmaceuticals and psychotropics as solutions.

Medicalization and pharmaceuticalization often refer to the reduction of complex, multicausational social problems into simplistic corporeal ones. Addiction and drug abuse are two such problems that lie at the intersection of both medicalization and pharmaceuticalization.

These two processes establish health care, pharmaceutical companies, and the criminal legal system as the arbiters of legal and healthy substance use and as the sources of treatment for illegal and unhealthy use. And yet, many of the very substances that are outlawed or identified as the source of addiction are produced by intensifying medicalization and pharmaceuticalization processes that are substantially funded and supported by laboratories, legislation, and discourse produced and supported by the state.

A central mechanism of biopower is the successful internalization of an individualized civic duty to live long, healthy, productive lives.[42] It requires believing in and living a life aligned with the scientific discourse and expertise that dictate acceptable and desirable ways of being. In so doing, individuals need not be diagnosed, policed, or labeled by medicine or the carceral system, as they do this work all on their own. They *aspire* to be their "best self": wealthy, healthy, fertile, self-sufficient, and productive, which just so happens to conform to the images put forth by these dominant institutions. In accordance with these aspirations, power is rendered invisible as it is experienced productively: *inspiring* individuals to behave in certain ways, rather than threatening them.

This neoliberal imperative directs attention away from institutions and practices that effectively *maim* individuals, thwarting their productive efforts. In her book *The Right to Maim: Debility, Capacity, Disability*, queer theorist Jasbir Puar disrupts the traditional binary between ability and disability by asking us to interrogate the relationship between disability, capacity, and *debility*. She asks us to consider how "some bodies may not be recognized as or identify as disabled," despite being "debilitated, in part by being foreclosed access to legibility and resources as disabled."[43] For example, those who are raised in underfunded school districts may be debilitated in terms of their educational resources. However, they are not recognized as disabled in the traditional sense as their disadvantage is structural rather than biological. Rather than biological features of the body, debility and capacity are the direct result of institutional (mis)recognition and structural in- or exclusivity. This explains why "some bodies may well be disabled but also capacitated,"[44] such as those with recognized learning disabilities that result in institutional accommodation. Many bodies are debilitated by our culture but are not recognized as disabled and therefore receive neither individual- nor group-level accommodations, nor do they mobilize collective effort for structural change.

Such debilitation has resulted in underfunded and overpoliced communities that increasingly feel more like prisons themselves. The lines between prison and such communities are increasingly blurred and have resulted in what sociologist Loïc Wacquant has termed a "carceral continuum."[45] This term refers to the increasingly formalized carceral net that entangles more and more people under the guise of diversion or rehabilitation. As sociologist Kerwin Kaye argues in *Enforcing Freedom*, the entire model of therapeutic jurisprudence, including drug courts, is to eradicate the "drugs lifestyle" and prepare marginalized populations for low-wage labor and further exploitation and systemic abuse. Many who find themselves ensnared in the carceral system of drug courts, mandated rehabilitation programs, supervision, and parole often have only minimal involvement with substances yet have been deemed to be *at risk*—locating the problem in the body and the brain rather than the environment. Accordingly, the solution is "rehabilitation" of the individual psyche rather than addressing the "host of social and political problems—unemployment, housing instability, hunger, race and class discrimination, barriers to education, police harassment, among many others."[46] It also fails to account for the fact that the same individuals who are more likely to have problems medicalized and treated with drugs under a state surveillance program are also more likely to have that substance use criminalized and punished through the carceral system.

Prescription drugs exist at the liminal space between the *productive* and the *at risk*. When one follows the direction of a doctor, prescription drug use is productive. When undertaken independently, it is risky. While the risk is argued to be epidemiological (impact on one's health), in practice, the risk is institutional (arrest or incarceration).

Stratification via Criminalization

For the first three-quarters of the twentieth century, the prison population remained stable in the United States; on average, 110 out of 100,000 people were incarcerated each year. But those numbers started to increase in the 1970s, doubling in the 1980s, and doubling again in the 1990s. In 2018, 706 people were incarcerated out of 100,000, almost seven times the rate of 1900–1975.[47] Today, even though the United States is home to only 5 percent of the world population, it has over 20 percent of the world's incarcerated population. This is, in part, the result of legislation passed in the 1980s that established more stringent sentencing for drug-related offenses. Between 1982 and 1994, federal murder sentences decreased by almost 30 percent while drug sentences increased by 45 percent; state-level trends were similar. These laws and policies resulted in a 126 percent increase in drug arrests over the decade, resulting in a prison population larger than anywhere else in the world. This has become so extreme that sociologist Randall Shelden argues that "it has become progressively more serious to have been caught with drugs than to kill someone."[48]

These policies laid the foundation for what came to be termed the War on Drugs. This "war" was waged by the United States federal government on psychoactive drugs and those who used and distributed them. This was made possible by rendering drugs and people who used or distributed them as dangerous to the social body. Legislation shifted the focus from drug kingpins to low-level drug offenders. This resulted in an increase in policing, given the greater number of potential arrestees, but also resulted in their greater visibility, facilitating identification, arrest, and prosecution, all of which were financially and politically encouraged by the federal government. Drug crimes were increasingly punished with incarceration rather than probation and the length of sentences skyrocketed. The average length of incarceration jumped 153 percent between 1988 and 2012.[49]

The War on Drugs was racialized from the start. Drug policy, in tandem with policing and incarceration practices and the disenfranchisement of incarcerated people in the United States, has reentrenched the racial caste system that was previously upheld by the Atlantic slave trade and, later, Jim Crow segregationist policies. While drug laws do not explicitly mention race, in practice, they result in the disproportionate incarceration of African Americans, relegating them to a permanent second-class status where they are denied the very rights won by the civil rights movement, such as the right to vote, to serve on juries, and to be protected from discrimination in employment, housing, education, and securing social services.[50] This is made possible by the many wires of the "birdcage" of structural racism, including sentencing disparities, mandatory minimums, "zero tolerance" policies, all-white juries, and so-called colorblind algorithmic surveillance and policing systems that disproportionately target, arrest, and incarcerate Black and Brown communities.[51]

In recent years, mass incarceration has become increasingly diverse. This is not the result of declining incarceration rates among Black and Latinx individuals; instead, it reflects the influx of white prisoners. Civil rights activist and legal scholar Michelle Alexander terms the increasing incarceration of white people by a drug war designed to target Black and Brown people as "collateral damage." As she argues, "In any war, a tremendous amount of collateral damage is inevitable. Black and brown people are the principal targets in this war; white people are collateral damage." Alexander explains, "Saying that white people are collateral damage may sound callous, but it reflects a particular reality." It also allows for the veil of colorblindness to remain over the criminal legal system, whereby not *all* people behind bars are Black or Latinx, just the disproportionate majority.[52]

The influx of prisoners, many of whom are white, for the nonmedical use of prescription drugs reflects collateral damage. This book focuses on the criminalization of prescription drug use as an example of (1) the ever-widening net of carceral control, and (2) how quickly legislation might change to focus on rehabilitation rather than punishment when the majority of those who are impacted are increasingly white. It also draws attention to this issue as (3) nonmedical prescription drug use and overdose by prescription drugs are increasingly impacting Black and Latinx communities as well. While punishment for illicit substance use was designed to target people of color, access to prescription drugs (often of greater potency than street drugs) has been shaped by white privilege. The convergence of the medical and carceral systems initially impacted those at their nexus—poor, white communities—but in recent years it has extended its reach well beyond these bounds. Specifically, while initial rates of use and overdose of opioids were higher among white populations who had greater access to medical care and therefore to the prescriptions, rates of overdose for Black and Latinx individuals have skyrocketed in recent years, with some estimates showing a 40 percent increase between 2018 and 2019, so that now rates of overdose are comparable between white, Black, and Latinx individuals.[53]

Medicine and the criminal legal system exert social control through systems of classification that simultaneously allow and encourage the behaviors of some groups and deny and punish the behaviors of others. In doing so, they regulate social morality by designating certain acts illegal, thereby warranting punishment, while deeming certain acts a sign of sickness, warranting treatment.[54] Prescription drugs have become a technology of both institutions as they are simultaneously used to treat sickness and moderate criminality under a single moral economy where the boundary between treatment and punishment is often indistinguishable, such as prisons that heavily medicate institutionalized populations or court-mandated drug treatment programs that employ punishment as a form of treatment.[55] These interrelated systems of medicalization, pharmaceuticalization, and criminalization come together to form a prescription-to-prison pipeline.

The Prescription-to-Prison Pipeline: Where Medicalization and Criminalization Meet

The term *prescription-to-prison pipeline* draws upon a number of pipeline systems and concepts, including the Drug Enforcement Administration's Operation Pipeline, which was part of the Reagan administration's War on Drugs, as well as the *school-to-prison pipeline*, which described the strong association between children who have been removed from schools and subsequent incarceration.

Operation Pipeline was a federal program administered by over three hundred state and local law enforcement agencies to train law enforcement officers to use traffic stops as a pretext to search for drugs and use the drugs as the basis for arrest and prosecution.[56] While the program focused particularly upon traffic violations, the "volume" approach to law enforcement has come to include many other minor infractions, such as loitering, jaywalking, or appearing "suspicious," as defined by a law enforcement officer. While the proportion of searches that yield discovery of illegal substances is low, the logic assumes that more stops eventually result in more arrests.

The school-to-prison pipeline refers to the fact that children who are suspended or expelled from school are disproportionately Black, Latinx, poor, or have a documented disability, and that being removed from school in early childhood increases the likelihood of future incarceration.[57] Although schools claim to be "colorblind" in suspension or expulsion policies, Black students are suspended or expelled at a rate three times higher than white students. This trend begins as early as preschool, where almost half of children suspended or expelled before the age of five are Black.[58] As a result of "zero tolerance" policies, children who are suspended, expelled, or otherwise "pushed out" out of the school system are more likely to end up on the street, in the juvenile justice system, or in adult jails and prisons.[59] In fact, young Black men between the ages of twenty and twenty-four who do not have a high school diploma (or GED) have a greater chance of being incarcerated than of being employed.[60] The inverse relationship between education and incarceration is further revealed by the fact that 41 percent of those in prison did not complete high school, and the average offender reads at an eighth-grade level.[61] Despite this documented relationship, prison spending in the United States has increased at triple the rate that funding for public elementary and secondary education has.[62] Together, these data illustrate how disparities in funding, discipline, and education can create disparities in policing and incarceration, disproportionately impacting certain communities and individuals over others.

The prescription-to-prison pipeline refers to a similar relationship between communities that receive the least funding and support for quality health care, education, housing, employment, and nourishing environments while facing some of the highest levels of state surveillance, intervention, and control. Health care—including mental health support—is not a constitutional right in the United States. Instead, it is something that has historically been available to those with salaried jobs. As a result, those with inconsistent employment or wage-labor positions often experience fractured and incomplete health-care coverage and support. Sporadic interactions with health-care professionals can result in dangerous combinations of too-much and too-little medical intervention; this is exacerbated by the fact that psychotropics are increasingly prescribed by a wide range of health practitioners, rather than being prescribed by psychiatrists who have medical training and knowledge of substance effects.[63] Increasingly, psychotropics are prescribed without a psychiatric diagnosis. One study found that over 60 percent of visits where a new psychotropic was prescribed did not involve a psychiatric diagnosis.[64] These trends intersect in dangerous ways for those who receive health care as a part of state-mandated care (e.g., foster care, juvenile detention, school counselors, prisons), as medication regimens may be unjustified or uninterrogated. As sociologist Anthony Hatch asks, "What is the boundary between benevolent medicine and malevolent drugging?"[65] The prescription of drugs is always about control, but the question is: Who is the subject and object of that control?

Individuals with less power, specifically those with fewer financial, social, or cultural resources to direct, negotiate, or challenge their treatment, are especially vulnerable to medicine and prisons as twin institutions of control. In fact, administration of psychotropic drugs is the most common and often the only form of mental health care that incarcerated populations receive, sometimes accounting for more of a prison's budget than food.[66] And those subject to incarceration are disproportionately those who come from underresourced communities and families. Adults who live below the poverty line are three times more likely to be arrested than those above, and those earning less than 150 percent of the federal poverty level are fifteen times more likely to be charged with a felony than those above the poverty level.[67] Education is highly correlated with income; therefore it is no surprise that individuals with college education also receive shorter sentences than individuals without.[68] How exactly psychotropics are prescribed by state-enforced institutionalized settings exists in a black box, so it is impossible to fully understand, evaluate, or change the practice.[69] Unlike surveys that trace the use of psychotropics in noninstitutionalized settings, surveys about psychotropic prescription in prisons are administered infrequently, ask questions in different ways on each administration, and do not ask whether prisoners have been forced to take medications against their will—details that negate the possibility for a historical comparative analysis. Hatch argues that this obfuscation is intentional, hiding the ways in which prisons use psychotropics to control incarcerated populations.[70] He argues that many are forced to take these medications in the absence of formal diagnoses, and that "psychotropics are a major element of the policy approach called *technocorrections*, the strategic application of new technologies in the effort to reduce the costs of mass incarceration and minimize the risks that prisoners pose to society."[71] In other words, the United States would not be capable of incarcerating as many people as it does without psychotropics as a fundamental technology of the carceral system.

The prescription-to-prison pipeline refers to the ways that medicalization and pharmaceuticalization, both inside and outside of institutionalized settings, contribute to incarceration and recidivism among already underserved and overpoliced populations. It includes a wide range of interrelated structures, policies, and discourses that funnel certain groups and individuals into the carceral system. It includes people who were prescribed and used medication for a long duration before having their script abruptly discontinued and being forced to find alternative sources or ways to manage symptoms of withdrawal. It includes people who have experienced trauma and abuse, who were taught to manage their pain pharmacologically but were later criminalized for that same behavior. It includes people who work for meager wages, who began to use prescription drugs without a prescription as a way to self-medicate, to perform on the job, or to hold families together in the face of compounding injustices. It includes children separated from their families at a young age who were medicated for behavioral issues rather than being treated for trauma or reunited with families, only to have harms further compounded when they are criminalized for using those prescriptions in alternative ways. It includes all of these groups and others who have had social, political, and financial problems medicalized directly by health-care practitioners or more broadly by neoliberal, biomedical discourses but who as a consequence of their social location were subjected to greater carceral scrutiny and punishment. The prescription-to-prison pipeline refers to ways that criminalization *and* medicalization are used to reframe social and political problems such as unemployment, housing insecurity, family separation, and other forms of discrimination as *moral* and *biological* problems of substance abuse, addiction, or impulse control. It also justifies an increase in spending on corrections and psychotropic prescriptions and a reduction of spending on education, hospitals and health care, and public welfare.[72]

Hatch argues that the state asserts custodial power through the medicalization and (forcible) administration of psychotropics when it is deemed to be "in the best interest of the prisoner."[73] However, there are many people outside of institutionalized settings who use prescription drugs of their own volition to enact idealized behaviors or identities, because they believe these drugs will make them healthy or make them a "better version" of themselves, without realizing how these versions of themselves are those that help sustain existing (stratified) structures of society. This is able to occur in a society where the treatment of one's prescription drug use by institutions of control is not consistent. While some people's use of prescription drugs confers greater privilege and status (e.g., job promotion), others are further marginalized and oppressed (e.g., incarceration).

Prescription drugs may intensify existing axes of stratification. As is true for all interactions with the carceral system, those arrested or prosecuted for nonmedical prescription drug use are not all treated alike. Treatment by the criminal legal system remains stratified by race, class, and gender. While some are *blamed* for their *abuse* of drugs and told to take responsibility for the associated adverse outcomes, others are viewed as *victims* of the substances, doctors, or adverse situations that precipitated substance use. This is most apparent in the arrest and sentencing disparities between prescription opioids and cocaine. Despite the fact that prescription opioids have greater potential for overdose, there were nearly four times as many arrests for cocaine than for opioids in 2016, and individuals found guilty of cocaine-related charges are more often sentenced to prison, whereas those charged with opioid-related offenses are more likely to be sent to inpatient rehabilitation or therapeutic communities, as directed by drug courts. Black people were also more than three times as likely as white people to be arrested on charges related to heroin, opioids, and cocaine in 2016.[74] This reflects persistent racialized disparities in legislation, policing, and sentencing. As such, the harms of these systems remain stratified by race, class, and gender.

The People behind the Numbers and Labels

This book demonstrates that the boundaries between the medical and carceral systems, use and abuse, prescription and illicit drugs, productivity and pleasure, and physical and psychological pain are far more permeable than they are often presented as being but are preserved to justify medical and legal regulation. These binaries can be used to justify unequal treatment of drug use and maintain systems of control, legitimating the authority of medicine, doctors, and the law to regulate behavior and sort actors into hospitals, homes, or prisons.

This research aims to highlight how the relationship between pain, substance use, treatment, and incarceration is mediated by one's identities. Although data on substance use or incarceration, as presented by the National Institute on Drug Abuse (NIDA) or the Department of Justice (DOJ), are often spliced by singular identities such as sex, race, or age, the individuals behind those numbers are shaped by multiple, co-constitutive, identities. For example, it is not particularly meaningful to say that 50 percent of individuals who use prescription drugs are white if we do not know their other identity characteristics, such as gender, class, and education level, but also if we do not know their life histories. Did they experience trauma or abuse? Did they experience an injury or surgery that resulted in chronic pain? Were they diagnosed (or undiagnosed) with a mental health disorder? Were they in a high-pressure environment with limited social support? In other words, what were the contextual and personal factors that might help us understand why they used prescription drugs nonmedically and what were the subsequent factors that resulted in their incarceration?

Rather than thinking about race, class, and gender as a set of freestanding identities, intersectionality pushes us to interrogate how racism, (hetero)sexism, ageism, nationalism, neocolonialism, neoliberalism, and capitalism structure our experiences, often in mutually intensifying ways.[75] The emphasis upon structures and processes that influence how bodies and behaviors are experienced and treated differently draws attention to the fact that the meanings of identities are socially constructed rather than being biological realities.[76] Without such emphasis, it is easy for disparities along such demographic variables to be interpreted as the result of biological propensities to behave differently, rather than differential treatment by social institutions and individuals. So long as race, gender, and other social constructs continue to be treated as objective biological facts rather than social inventions, they may continue to be used to justify inequalities in medicine, housing, education, social class, and the criminal legal system rather than to interrogate how those institutions are *producing* those inequalities.[77] As author Ta-Nehisi Coates argues, "Race is the child of racism, not its father."[78]

While racism, classism, sexism, homophobia, and other forms of discrimination impact one's experiences of pain, medicalization, and overdose, these do not occur in uniform ways. While white, middle-class or affluent women may be more likely to be prescribed pills than men, other women are not. But there are also plenty of white, affluent women who are not prescribed pills—those who have been labeled an "addict," "hysterical," "weak," or "strong." In our personal lives, we recognize that we, our friends, and our family are not reducible to a series of demographic labels; our lives defy such reductionist explanations. However, institutions that survey and collect data on our life experiences, such as prescribing rates, substance use, and overdose, continue to do so in ways that reify these categories and potentially reverse causal arguments that interpret disparities as the outcome of some biological reality rather than the justification for racial classification. The self-reported race, gender, and age of respondents are included in this book because individuals are treated differently as a result of discrimination on the basis of perceived identities. However, these details should be treated as contextual information in understanding the life stories of the individuals in this book. My goal is to examine why certain bodies and populations are at greater risk of being medicalized, criminalized, or both. It is not the intention to locate this risk in bodies or populations themselves, but to draw attention to the structural violence that produces such inequities.

This book draws upon eighty interviews, each an hour long, conducted with people currently incarcerated in Missouri for a variety of charges (e.g., illicit drugs, theft, forgery, or homicide).[79] It draws upon the perspectives of the incarcerated in part because they are simultaneously invisible and hypervisible in society, but also because they are trapped in this nexus of increasing medication and regulation. It also centers the voices of those omitted from most nationally representative studies of drug use. For example, the National Institute on Drug Abuse (NIDA) and the Substance Abuse and Mental Health Services Administration (SAMHSA) have measured the severity of nonmedical prescription drug use in terms of overdose incidence. These data, while purportedly nationally representative, do not sample from institutionalized populations such as those in prisons or treatment centers. As a result, nonmedical prescription drug use—most often referred to by these agencies as "prescription drug misuse" or "abuse"—is considered a problem only insofar as it contributes to drug overdose. Such formulation casts the issue in limited terms, measuring consequences exclusively in terms of overdose numbers but also locating the cause of the problem in the drug or the individual using the drug rather than in the social and political environment that created the initial untreated pain.

While each of the issues has been explored separately—the medicalization of everyday life, how medical and carceral systems work together to control populations, the impacts of therapeutic jurisprudence, factors that have contributed to rises in opioid use and overdose, and how the War on Drugs has institutionalized racism, classism, and sexism[80]—this book brings into focus how these processes work together to produce a prescription-to-prison pipeline. Building upon the work of these scholars, I tease out the multiple factors that motivate nonmedical prescription drug use, the stratified treatment of that use, and the broader structural and institutional factors that construct the meanings of *nonmedical use, substance abuse, addiction*, and the *user* or *addict* that similarly distract us from place and context by focusing on individual willpower, brain science, and chemical compounds. Further, I draw attention to how such discourses are rendered "colorblind" while simultaneously contributing to racial disparities in treatment and outcomes. In so doing, I highlight how colorblind racism plays a central role in how similar situations of substance use are treated differently by medicine, science, and the law.[81] I show this by adopting an intersectional approach that takes into consideration interviewees' different social identities and how social locations impact how those identities are treated. As much as possible, I situate their perspectives in relationship to personal life experiences and structural conditions that shape how they perceive and interact with both medical and carceral systems.

This book centers the perspectives of the incarcerated, given that they are one of the most marginalized populations. In her book *Are Prisons Obsolete?*, revolutionary philosopher Angela Davis critiques the US criminal justice system, arguing that the prison has come to function "ideologically as an abstract site into which undesirables are deposited, relieving us of the responsibility of thinking about the real issues afflicting those communities from which prisoners are drawn in such disproportionate numbers." In doing so, "it relieves us of the responsibility of seriously engaging with the problems of our society, especially those produced by racism and, increasingly, global capitalism."[82] This has increasingly become the case with the nonmedical use of prescription drugs.

The experiences of the incarcerated affect us all. Almost half of all people living in the United States have experienced the incarceration of a parent, spouse, sibling, or child. More than five million children in the United States have had a parent incarcerated. Forty-five percent of men aged twenty-four or younger in state or federal prisons are fathers, and 48 percent of women in federal prison, and 55 percent in state facilities, are mothers. In the state of Missouri, 7 percent of children (98,000 children) have grown up with an incarcerated parent.[83] Black adults are twice as likely as white adults to have an immediate family member incarcerated, and those relatives are three times more likely to be imprisoned for over a year. Latinx individuals are 70 percent more likely than white individuals to be locked up for more than a year.[84]

As harrowing as the national statistics are, trends in Missouri, where the vast majority of the people interviewed grew up, are even worse. Missouri has the eighth highest incarceration rate out of the fifty US states. Rates of juvenile custody are also higher in Missouri than the average juvenile custody rates in the United States. Specifically, Missouri has the seventeenth highest juvenile custody rate out of the fifty US states.[85] Further, Missouri has the fourth highest prescribing rate of benzodiazepines (e.g., Xanax, Klonopin, and Valium).[86] This is particularly concerning given that before August 2021, Missouri was the only state that did not enforce a federal law designed to ensure mental health care is covered by insurance providers at the same rate as physical ailments. Relatedly, Missouri has one of the most acute shortages of mental health specialists,[87] since many of them were not reimbursed the same way they might be in other states. This only exacerbates the situation of a health-care system where the majority of psychotropics are prescribed by primary care doctors.[88] If we look beyond mood stabilizers, in 2012, Missouri averaged 95.4 opioid prescriptions per 100 people,[89] and until 2021, Missouri remained the only state without a prescription drug monitoring system. These are some of the many reasons why this research focuses on the state of Missouri, given that national trends were even more acute at the state level.

It is not the intention of this book to vilify or exalt any individuals, groups, or institutions over others. Instead, I seek to present the experiences and interpretations from the perspectives of my interviewees and provide a historical and institutional context for such claims. Many interviewees have caused harm to themselves or to others. They described such incidents, for which they felt guilt or shame. However, they were also often victims of considerable harms over their lifetimes. And in many cases, they did not recognize that their experiences were traumatic or that they were not responsible for them. While I do not seek to absolve anyone from responsibility for their actions (nor do I have the power to do so), I also draw attention to broader punitive discourses that cause these individuals to assume full culpability given that they are often trapped at the nexus of intersecting forms of inequality.

While the majority of the people interviewed for this project came from hardship or poverty, or experienced considerable trauma and abuse, it is important to note that the majority of people who experience these things do not end up using prescription drugs nonmedically and do not become incarcerated. Further, many people who use prescription drugs nonmedically do not come from the same type of hardship—in fact, many come from relative privilege, and yet they do not suffer the impacts of medicalization and criminalization of their substance use that our interviewees did.

There is an important interplay between structure and agency that is illustrated by these stories, as there is in all our lives. It is not the intention of this book to portray people as lacking that agency or to imply that their life outcomes are overdetermined, but rather to identify and trace institutional structures and cultural discourses that may limit how events, technologies, and behaviors are interpreted. The goal is to help identify the actual problems at play and some tenable solutions.

Organization of the Book

This book argues that the medicalization of endemic social problems in tandem with the criminalization of those problems and their medical solutions exacerbates inequality along lines of race, class, and gender and expands the carceral net. Although not all trajectories progress in the same linear fashion, as people enter the pipeline at different stages, many experience each stage of this process at some point as the circuit becomes recursive and totalizing. There-fore, each chapter of this book traces one element of this process. Chapter 1, "The Medicalization and Criminalization of Pain," begins with a discussion of pain itself. Only in recent history has pain been considered to be a medi-cal ailment in and of itself warranting medical and pharmaceutical interven-tion. The medicalization of pain narrows the scope of prevention or treatment to the corporeal level and blinds us to the structural factors that could wield much greater influence than a tiny (though mighty) pill. Seeing how pain it-self is unevenly distributed in the population makes evident that pain is not an individual-level problem but rather a social one. Situating the medicalization of pain in the broader political and social history of substance use and regu-lation in the United States, we see how medicalization and criminalization are unevenly patterned across groups in the United States, which entrenches existing axes of inequality. As a consequence, privileged groups and entities are protected from control or punishment for their substance use, whereas marginalized groups are perpetually at risk of having their actions criminal-ized. Such protection and prosecution are facilitated in large part by legislation that has shielded pharmaceutical companies, doctors, and the well-resourced from serious legal consequences while simultaneously criminalizing marginal-ized communities and communities of color and legalizing surveillance ter-rorism of these groups. In recent years, such stratification has been intensified by the medicalization of substance use and abuse. Countering the assumption that health-care providers, treatment, and rehabilitation centers offer alterna-tives to penal institutions, this chapter outlines the ways in which they extend and intensify a carceral net that surveils, controls, and punishes and that does little to address pain or adverse outcomes of substance use, but rather increases their incidence.

Chapter 2, "Prescription: Getting Hooked," explores how the overreliance upon pharmacological solutions often exacerbates endemic social problems such as pov-erty, gender inequality, abuse, and trauma. Both pain and health care are unequally distributed in US society, and those without access to broader financial, social, and political support systems are more likely to be treated with a prescription pad. This chapter presents the stories of interviewees who were prescribed opi-oids to manage pain associated with injuries incurred on the job or as a result of violence; psychotropics to deal with childhood abuse, trauma, or hardship; or opioids and psychotropics to assist with pregnancy, childbirth, or early moth-erhood. Many interviewees were taught early on to medicate their problems, a practice that later resulted in arrest and imprisonment. Their experiences reflect the broader neoliberal imperative and medicalization of society, but also how this medicalization intersects with criminalization for those who are subject to greater surveillance. This chapter draws attention to systems of marginalization that were intensified by medicalization processes.

Chapter 3, "Pipeline: Sorting Use from Abuse," explores how the sorting and labeling processes involved in policing prescription drugs initiate and perpetuate systems of inequality. Despite the biological language of substance abuse or addiction as a "brain disease," diagnostic criteria of such "disorders" are behavioral and directly linked to existing socioeconomic and social structures, such as one's performance on the job or at school. As a consequence, failure to contribute to a capitalist, neoliberal economy has been transformed into a symptom of addiction or a substance use disorder, warranting medical or carceral intervention. The chapter explores how the regulation of substance use has been tied to the regulation of a race-, class-, and gender-based social structure. In doing so, it highlights how medical practitioners have worked alongside and via the criminal legal system to pathologize substance use for some groups, while simultaneously encouraging substance use among others. Such pathologization most often takes the form of diagnostic and judicial labels such as "addicts" and "criminals," which result in restrictions and heightened surveillance and the increased likelihood of eventual incarceration. Interviewees' stories reveal how medicine and prisons work together to monitor, diagnose, and manage individuals in ways that result in perpetual medical-penal surveillance and, for the already marginalized, the prescription-to-prison pipeline.

Chapter 4, "Prison: From Medicalization to Criminalization," explores how the prescription-to-prison pipeline has contributed to the net-widening effects of the carceral system. Through the experiences of those whose substance use has been medicalized and criminalized, it becomes evident how treatment and incarceration are two sides of the same coin that seeks to control, surveil, and punish those who do not behave or present themselves the way that society has deemed appropriate. While holistic health care can advantage those already advantaged by race, class, and gender, the marginalized may find their situations only made worse through the medicalization process that extends carceral surveillance, control, and punishment.

Contrary to the popular narrative that drug use, poverty, violence, and incarceration are the result of individual choices or biological deficits, this book demonstrates that these social problems are the product of environmental and structural factors, including underfunded school systems, unlivable wages, incompatibility of work and childcare schedules and costs, stratified policing, and overreliance upon pharmacological solutions to social, financial, and political problems. The adverse effects of substance use are tied to a stark divide in income and wealth in this country, a divide that is directly linked to inequities in health care, education, policing, and incarceration as well as discrimination along lines of race, class, and gender. The conclusion to this book, "When Medicine Becomes a Drug," interrogates how medicalization practices exacerbate preexisting inequalities and have contributed to the prescription-to-prison pipeline, while offering policy solutions and counternarratives. The proposed solutions are broad and far-reaching, given that the prescription-to-prison-pipeline is overdetermined by many interlocking structural factors related to employment, health care, social support, policing, and the political and social economy. In this book, I outline the multiple overlapping and multidirectional ways by which individuals are funneled into the pipeline. Although the title implies a singular pipeline and process, there are multiple avenues by which someone may get pulled or pushed into the system. Once they are inside, marked by negative medical and legal credentials,[90] it becomes increasingly challenging to escape.

If, as a society, the United States decided to invest in the social services to assist individuals with health care, counseling, employment, and housing, as opposed to more "quick fixes" such as pharmaceutical drugs and prisons, perhaps it could disrupt the prescription-to-prison pipeline, as well as reduce adverse effects associated with substance use and incarceration. Lyndsey did not want to go to prison. She didn't want to hurt her children. She didn't want to spend her life in pursuit of more drugs, only to feel relief for just a short while. She wants to spend time with her children, find steady employment and housing to support them, and have some time to herself every once in a while. But sometimes she feels as though the system is rigged against her. And maybe it is.

I

THE MEDICALIZATION AND
CRIMINALIZATION OF PAIN

In 1980, the World Health Organization declared that "freedom from pain" was a universal human right.[1] Pharmaceutical companies, particularly in the United States, capitalized upon this promise, offering patients chemical solutions to physical, emotional, and environmental problems. This effort proved successful. Of those surveyed between 2015 and 2016, almost half (45.8 percent) had used a prescription drug in the past thirty days.[2] Individuals have increasingly learned to cope with social problems through medical technologies such as prescription drugs.

Pain continues to be a significant health issue and health-care challenge in the United States. An estimated one in six men and one in five women experience pain on any given day.[3] In 1995, pain was adopted by health-care providers as the "fifth vital sign," measuring pain on a numerical scale alongside blood pressure, heart rate, respiratory rate, and temperature. The pain scale was added to both health assessments and patient satisfaction surveys. Treating pain as an ailment in and of itself rather than a mere symptom allowed doctors to legally—and liberally—prescribe opioids for chronic pain or for recovery from surgery or accidents. The goal was to improve pain care for patients with both chronic and acute pain.

Asking patients to rate their pain on a numerical scale presumes that it serves as a consistent measure of somatosensory pain. Contrary to this assumption, research indicates that these scores reflect emotional qualities of pain more than sensory intensity. Patients rate their pain considerably higher if they are anxious, depressed, fearful, or angry.[4] This is significant given that patients who rate their pain higher on the scale tend to be prescribed opioids at higher rates. In fact, one study suggests that anxiety and depression are inadvertently treated with opiates because these conditions can amplify physical pain as measured by this scale.[5]

This unidimensional, numerical scale for pain measurement sought to standardize treatment, a purpose similar to that of the other four vital signs: blood pressure, pulse rate, respiratory rate, and temperature. Reliance on these measurements assumes that human bodies conform to the same standards and that those that do not conform to these standards are necessarily sick and require medical intervention. Yet, as is true with the other four vital signs, pain is also context- and person-dependent.

However, unlike the other four vital signs, which can be measured by doctors, the pain scale is evaluated by the patient, thereby shifting the balance of power between the doctor and patient, if their patient were to be trusted and believed. Tipping the scales even further, pain-focused questions were included in patient satisfaction surveys, whereby patients could rate health-care providers negatively if their pain went untreated. In recent years, patient satisfaction surveys have become tied to state and federal funding (e.g., Medicare and Medicaid), thereby incentivizing hospitals and doctors to increase patient satisfaction scores. One way to increase patient satisfaction is to treat pain as quickly as possible, often with a prescription pad.[6]

In 2016, the American Medical Association voted to stop treating pain as the fifth vital sign, arguing that it may have contributed to increases in opioid overdose.[7] However, it was not replaced with an alternative strategy for dealing with the ongoing health issue of chronic pain. It also reaffirmed a power structure between health-care providers and patients—providers rather than patients have access to medical knowledge as captured by thermometers, blood pressure cuffs, and pulse oximeters and the medical credentials that permit interpretation and treatment. Physical and psychological pain remain significant public health crises that cannot be objectively measured by technologies (although the previously listed technologies also vary considerably based on contextual factors) and are often treated by the medical establishment only at the self-reported symptom level. While the more affluent are more likely to have access to long-term, consistent, and holistic treatment and to be believed by health-care professionals, the majority of Americans struggle to coordinate their care between a range of specialists as their story and symptoms get lost and questioned in an extensive game of telephone. This can result in redundant or insufficient treatment, both of which can produce deleterious outcomes.

The right to be free from pain is available only to those who are deemed responsible and suffering from legitimate pain and who agree to subject themselves to regular legal-medical surveillance.[8] Individuals who are not believed or who are deemed untrustworthy may be labeled "addicts" or "criminals" and thereby stripped of these rights *and* increasingly surveilled and controlled, sometimes through even greater medication.[9] The regulation of substance use, including prescription drugs, has also always been about regulating morality, respectability, class, race, and gender. Individuals who use substances must be deemed responsible, morally fit, and productive members of society in order to avoid external controls of their behavior.[10]

By tracing the major institutions that have shaped beliefs on pain and medication, we can see how a paradigm of "just right" medication, which emerged amid a host of contradictory assumptions, definitions, and instructions, continues to promulgate a moral boundary between the legitimate, suffering patient and the conniving, hedonistic criminal. The power to define use or abuse rests in the hands of the elite—doctors, lawyers, and politicians—often resulting in a double standard that allows some groups to use substances more liberally without reprimand, while others face greater marginalization because of their use. It also demonstrates how the prescription-to-prison-pipeline is the product of a combination of under- and overtreatment among individuals who are structurally disadvantaged in ways that increase the likelihood and intensity of pain in the first place.

Inequality of Pain: Too Little Health Care,
Income, or Social Support

Pain is a political issue. It is also a social and economic one. When we debate who is deserving of disability benefits, we are often discussing pain. When legislators define who is deserving of rent control protections or a restraining order, albeit rarely discussed explicitly, pain is a central consideration. What constitutes a living wage or fair trade designation is also about pain. Although rarely cast in such terms, effective social, political, and economic policies protect vulnerable populations from pain. As a result, they remain economic or political problems, while pain remains a medical problem. In siloing these interrelated, exacerbating processes, the solutions also remain disconnected.

This division is strategic. If pain is biomedical, then it is experienced at the individual level, its cause is internal rather than external, and the solution is pharmacological rather than political. Conceptualizing pain in this way minimizes or dismisses common pathways to pain—poverty, violence, or ineffective health care—and also impedes its treatment, which would benefit from social and political interventions rather than biomedical ones. In his book *Pain: A Political History*, historian Keith Wailoo chronicles how pain has become politicized in the United States. At the heart of this struggle is the concept of legitimacy: Which pain is legitimate, which is fraudulent, who is in genuine need of pain management, and who are drug seekers? This division between the deserving and undeserving reflects the politics of cultural citizenship policed by health practitioners, policy legislators, police officers, judges, and researchers and influenced by business interests.[11] As documented in books by two investigative journalists—Barry Meier's *Pain Killer* and Patrick Radden Keefe's *Empire of Pain*—pharmaceutical companies such as Purdue Pharma have persistently argued that "fraudulent users" are responsible for drug dependence, rather than aggressive marketing, liberal prescription, hyperpotency, or the absence of alternative forms of treatment and social support for those experiencing pain.[12]

One's race, class, gender, and age are significant in that they impact the likelihood that someone will experience pain, be prescribed medication, or be criminalized for nonmedical use. These factors contribute to one's broader social location, which determines access to health care, as well as school, employment opportunities, childcare, financial security, and other factors that contribute both to pain and to options for pain management.

Inequalities in pain are exacerbated by inequalities in health care. Low-income households are less likely to receive quality medical care than middle- and high-income households.[13] They are less likely to be insured, to have paid sick leave or parental leave, or to have the ability to take unpaid time off to make it to a doctor's office or hospital.[14] Recovering from an injury or illness is much more difficult without insurance, access to quality health care, reliable transportation, or paid sick leave. And without full recovery, pain begets pain.

Health care saves lives. Seeing a doctor in an emergency is important, but preventive medicine is more highly correlated with health and longevity.[15] Simply knowing that you have health insurance can significantly improve your self-reported health.[16] Unsurprisingly, access to quality health care and health insurance coverage is highly stratified along lines of class, but it is also stratified along divisions of race and ethnicity, which in turn impacts health outcomes.

Specifically, Black individuals are less likely to receive necessary health care for many reasons related to structural racism.[17] As a result of long-standing residential segregation and divestment, Black individuals are more likely to live in places with higher rates of pollution, violence, policing, and overcrowded housing, all of which impact one's health.[18] They are also less likely to have access to affordable healthy food, green spaces, and well-equipped and fully staffed hospitals and health-care centers.[19] Research indicates that the proportion of Black residents in a neighborhood is directly correlated with hospital closures.[20] In St. Louis, Missouri, this trend has been particularly acute: in 1970, the city had eighteen hospitals in predominantly Black neighborhoods, yet by 2010, all but one had shuttered, severely limiting health-care access.[21] These closures are compounded by "physician flight," whereby licensed health-care providers leave underfunded hospitals thereby intensifying health-care shortages.[22] Without access to primary care doctors, individuals in these communities are more likely to seek care in emergency rooms and public hospitals, which challenges efforts to provide consistent preventive care. Prior to the implementation of the Affordable Care Act in 2010, 32 percent of Latinx individuals were uninsured, as were 28 percent of Native Americans, and 21 percent of African Americans, compared to 13 percent of white individuals.[23]

Today, treatment remains stratified between those who receive government-sponsored health-care coverage and those who receive private coverage, which is patterned along racial lines due to persistent racial discrimination in the workplace as well as racial bias among health-care providers.[24] Surveys indicate that health-care providers continue to believe that Black and Latinx patients have a higher tolerance for pain and therefore treat ailments less aggressively, resulting in premature death.[25] Black and Indigenous women are three times as likely as white women to die during childbirth.[26] Lest we think this is an issue of class or education rather than race, we need only to look at the fact that college-educated Black women are five times as likely to die in childbirth as white women,[27] which makes it impossible to deny that Black patients continue to receive separate and unequal health care.

Black and Latinx patients wait much longer to receive medical care in hospitals, are more likely to have their intentions questioned, and are considerably less likely to receive pain medication.[28] On the surface, this last piece—receiving pain medication at lower rates—might appear to be positive, as the overdose crisis is often understood as the result of overmedication; however, this ignores the fact that Black, Indigenous, and Latinx patients are the least likely to receive preventive health care and mental health-care services or timely treatment, which contributes to pain, morbidity, and mortality.[29] Further, discrimination has been correlated with health metrics such as increased blood pressure as well as heightened risk of mortality.[30] Inequities in prescribing may also force individuals to seek alternative avenues or substances, which may be more potent or deadly. In other words, racism itself is a public health crisis. Such racial and ethnic inequities are further exacerbated by class inequality.

Inequalities in health care stem from and reflect the broader inequalities in US society. The gap between the rich and the poor has widened considerably over the last three decades. Since 1979, the income for the bottom fifth of earners—families earning less than $18,000 a year—has fallen a percentage point, while the top fifth's income has increased by 7 percent. The top 1 percent has seen gains of 6 percent of their income during this same time. In raw dollars, this means that the top fifth is earning, at minimum, an additional $25,000 each year, which is substantially more than what those in the bottom fifth earn *in total*.[31] This trend only worsened in recent years as a result of economic recessions. For example, after the economic downturn in 2008, low-wage workers struggled to find work. Industries shifted from coal to wind, from manufacturing jobs in Detroit to tech jobs in Silicon Valley. Factories moved abroad, and skills for employment shifted from building with machines to building with code. Technological advancements and the globalization of the world economy have contributed to job polarization where most job growth is concentrated either in high-skill, high-wage industries or low-skill, low-wage ones. The middle-skill, classic white-collar job disappeared.[32] This polarization has been further exacerbated by the decline in labor unions and changes to the tax system, which puts a greater proportional tax burden upon the poor than upon the rich.[33] During the COVID-19 pandemic in 2020, those who were able to keep their jobs and work from home disproportionately hailed from the middle and upper classes. As the unemployment numbers soared to the highest levels in almost a century, those who remained in the workforce were stratified into high-income jobs where most people could work from home and "essential" wage labor positions where individuals risked their lives by working in grocery stores, gas stations, and hardware stores.

Income inequality is particularly consequential in the United States, where society is predicated upon self-sufficiency at the nuclear family level. It is up to individual families to make it work. This is in contrast to other countries and cultures that take on a more communal approach to social support—broadening to the neighborhood, town, or even national level through both official and informal social safety nets, higher taxes paid by middle and upper classes, and providing other basic services to those in need. At a policy level, such services include generous parental leave policies, free or affordable child-care, school schedules that align with work schedules, and a mandated living wage. Culturally, it reflects communities in which children are raised collectively, where those who are sick, elderly, or unable to provide for themselves are cared for by others rather than being left to fend for themselves. It also reflects a health-care system that guarantees coverage for all.

The Power of Prescription: Protection from Regulation

Pain has become a disease to be treated in and of itself rather than the symptom of an unequal society. The proliferation of medication is often interpreted as an indication of scientific progress—that we are able to identify solutions to long-standing problems. However, this optimistic (and simplistic) explanation fails to consider that many prescriptions do not fix the underlying problems but instead distract us from them and can themselves create new ones. The discovery of morphine and opium are prime examples of this process.

Upon their discovery, doctors enthusiastically prescribed opium and morphine for a wide range of ailments. They were prescribed "to dull pain, induce sleep, control insanity, alleviate cough, check diarrhea, and treat a wide range of communicable diseases, including malaria, smallpox, syphilis, and tuberculosis."[34] It was not until caseloads of patients had already been prescribed and become dependent upon them that medical authorities became concerned about their addictive properties. But doctors were too reluctant to give up on one of their most powerful tools.

As opiates became the panacea for physical pain in the nineteenth and twentieth centuries, psychotropics have become the cure-all for psychic pain or mood regulation in the twenty-first. More than one in ten individuals in the United States are prescribed a psychotropic, including antidepressants, sedatives, and tranquilizers.[35] Between 2014 and 2016, the physician office visit rate at which benzodiazepines were prescribed was twenty-seven annual visits per one hundred adults, many of which were for chronic conditions, despite the fact these substances have not been designed for long-term use. Among visits at which benzodiazepines were prescribed, approximately one-third involved an overlapping opioid prescription, which can be potentially a lethal combination.[36]

The vast majority of antidepressants and other psychotropics are prescribed by nonpsychiatrists who are not properly trained to diagnose or treat mental health.[37] While their intentions are often to help patients in need, such prescriptions may cause more—rather than alleviate—harm. The health-care system in the United States is designed to promote this type of medical practice; while talk therapy is reimbursed by insurance companies at abysmally low rates and amounts, prescribing drugs or performing a medical procedure receives higher and more consistent compensation.[38]

Pharmaceutical companies have exacerbated this trend by promoting pharmaceutical solutions to anything deemed a social problem. In this context, the line between prescription drugs to treat ailments and those to enhance (e.g., Viagra) is increasingly blurred.[39] Of the most developed nations in the world, the United States has the most permissive environment for pharmaceutical companies, which is a major factor shaping the medicalization of social problems.

The proliferation of prescription drugs in the United States has been made possible, in part, by Direct-to-Consumer (DTC) and Direct-to-Prescriber (DTP) advertising as well as loosened regulation of the pharmaceutical industry. These three processes are directly linked. As chronicled in Patrick Radden Keefe's book *Empire of Pain*, the Sackler family of Purdue Pharma became notorious for all three. This was evidenced by the fact that Arthur Sackler, the eldest brother behind Purdue Pharma, was inducted into the Medical Advertising Hall of Fame with the declaration that "no single individual did more to shape the character of medical advertising" than he, as he brought "the full power of advertising and promotion to pharmaceutical advertising."[40] Focusing on both prescribers and patients, the Sackler family managed to both market and sell Valium and OxyContin at rates exceeding any previous tranquilizer or painkiller, respectively. Valium became the first $100 million drug in history, while OxyContin resulted in over $12 billion in revenue. This was the result of successful marketing and negotiation with doctors, as well as pressure upon regulatory bodies such as the Food and Drug Administration (FDA).[41]

As of 2020, the United States is one of only two countries that allow DTC marketing of prescription drugs on the television, in newspapers, in magazines, and on the internet,[42] allowing pharmaceutical companies to market directly to patients, who are, as a result, transformed into consumers. The impact of these regulations can be measured by the proliferation of these advertisements across US media. In 2017 alone, pharmaceutical companies spent $5.8 billion on DTC advertising.[43] Adjusting for inflation, that dollar amount is over fifteen times the amount spent in 1960, which was $2.6 million.[44] This turned out to be a good return on investment given that in 2018, Americans spent $360 billion on prescription drugs.[45]

Direct-to-Prescriber marketing is associated with increased prescribing behaviors of physicians, as well as increased rates of overdose by patients.[46] One study found that purchasing even a single meal with a value of twenty dollars for a doctor could be enough to change the way they prescribe.[47] Pharmaceutical companies such as Purdue Pharma spent millions of dollars each year just purchasing meals for physicians.[48] Limited regulation allowed such lobbying and aggressive marketing campaigns to both consumers and prescribers that misrepresented the addictive properties of drugs like OxyContin.[49] Just as the gun lobby in the United States argues that "guns do not kill people, people kill people," Purdue Pharma insisted that drugs such as Valium or OxyContin were not responsible for dependence, symptoms of withdrawal, or death: the source of the problem was the irresponsible *abusers* rather than the drugs themselves.[50] The same dollars that went to pressuring the FDA to expedite approval processes, lobbying the Drug Enforcement Administration to raise limits on the quota of oxycodone to be legally manufactured in the United States, and funding DTC and DTP marketing also contributed to media campaigns and lobbying efforts that constructed the problem as one of illicit abuse rather than of an unregulated substance or market. Thus users of the substances, rather than manufacturers, regulators, or prescribers, became the irresponsible actors in need of surveillance and punishment.[51]

Constructing the Racialized Addict: An Individual-Level Problem

While prescription drug companies and doctors have benefited from underregulation and legal protection, marginalized groups have suffered from overregulation and criminalization. In fact, the first law to exclude an entire ethnic group, the Chinese Exclusion Act of 1882, was passed in response to a carefully constructed moral panic that cast Chinese men as opium addicts whose substance use enabled them to steal jobs and women from white men. The legislation initially focused on the drug, using race-neutral language focused on protectionism and public health; however, as it evolved into the Chinese Exclusion Act, its racist and xenophobic intent became more readily apparent. And yet, through the criminalization of certain behaviors, racial inequities could be explained away as the result of individual choices rather than systemic discrimination.

As described in the previous section, the therapeutic use of opium had been common in colonial America and Europe. It was used to treat pain, cough, fever, and sleep disorders in addition to communicable diseases such as malaria and smallpox.[52] However, much like subsequent drug legislation in the United States, the prohibition of opium use or sale provided a colorblind mechanism for the exclusion and punishment of a social group—in this case, Chinese men.[53] Although many Chinese workers came to the United States as indentured laborers who hoped to pay off their debt quickly so they could return home to their families, they were constructed as a national threat to both the financial and moral economy of the country: profiting from railroad jobs and opium dens, while spreading addiction to vulnerable white women.[54] The combined efforts of the Chinese Exclusion Act of 1882 followed by the Geary Act of 1892 and a Supreme Court case in 1902 managed to ban Chinese immigration to the United States for almost sixty years. Further, in 1909, the import of opium to the United States from China was banned, thereby criminalizing the possession of opium for anyone who could not prove "to the satisfaction of a jury that they had it for legitimate reasons," which proved challenging for a person with Chinese ancestry standing in front of an all-white jury.[55] As medical historian David Musto argued, it was "the Southerner's fear of the Negro and the Westerner's fear of the Chinese" rather than concern about substance use that shaped American drug policy.[56]

While castigating opium dens as immoral and also illegal, middle-class white people increasingly frequented soda fountains at the turn of the twentieth century, enjoying *legal* beverages, such as Coca-Cola. In 1891, an Atlanta newspaper revealed what many of its consumers already knew: that Coca-Cola contained cocaine. However, the drug—and the soda—remained legal. It was only once Coca-Cola began to manufacture and distribute its product in glass bottles, thus "moving Coke out of the segregated space of the soda fountain," that "middle-class whites worried that soft drinks were contributing to what they saw as exploding cocaine use among African-Americans."[57] Motivated by racist fears of a mythical "Negro coke fiend,"[58] Coca-Cola removed cocaine from its product in 1903. Just as opium was outlawed as a means of regulating interracial relationships between Chinese men and white women, cocaine was outlawed in the Jim Crow South on the grounds that cocaine made Black men hypersexual and violent, causing them to rape white women and imbuing their bodies with superhuman strength, rendering them impervious to bullet wounds.[59] This controlling image of violent and sexual Black men was a means of transforming the notion of consensual interracial relationships into coercive and threatening ones, not unlike what was done to Chinese men.

The Ku Klux Klan had made similar arguments about the alcohol consumption of Catholics and immigrant working classes in their plea for a federal prohibition of alcohol around the same time. The criminalization of marijuana twenty years later would use the same recycled racist arguments about migrant Mexican farm workers in search of work.[60] In each of these instances, a controlling image of a subset of the population is constructed as a means of justifying legislation and the targeted punishment and control of a particular group.[61]

None of these racialized allegations were corroborated by evidence. In fact, contrary to the other popular narrative that opium use peaked among soldiers who self-medicated after the Civil War, data collected at the time suggest that substance use and dependence were most common among affluent, white women, who were barred from serving in the army but who were frequent subjects of the medical gaze.[62] Similar to upwardly mobile Chinese laborers or Black business owners, white women were viewed as threatening to the existing sociopolitical order. Therefore, while opium and morphine were regularly prescribed to white, affluent, American women to treat menstrual cramps, they were also prescribed to them for "anxiety," "hysteria," or "diseases of a nervous character."[63] Such diagnoses—made by white, upper-middle-class, male doctors—were often used to discredit or subdue "unruly" or "disruptive" women who sought equality or political power.

Men with the highest rates of opiate use were physicians themselves. At the time, 99 percent of all people addicted to morphine and opium had been prescribed these drugs by physicians; given that they were the population with the greatest power and access to these substances, it is no surprise that the prescribers were often using substances themselves.[64] What is significant is that affluent, white men and women who used opiates—both with and without a doctor's prescription—rarely experienced criminalization or medicalization in the form of labels such as "addiction."

In fact, elites in power crafted a different story: that nonwhite and low-income populations used substances more frequently than affluent, white populations. To justify policing efforts, a government campaign was launched to demonize the "Negro dope fiend," casting him as an immoral criminal who lacks self-control and makes no productive contributions to society. This caricature was based upon the early twentieth-century construction of the urban "junkie," shorthand for "junkman," who was most often white, male, and lower class. The term *junkie* emerged in the 1920s to describe a type of person in New York City who financed their drug supply by collecting scraps of copper, lead, zinc, and iron from industrial dumps and selling them to a dealer. The term gained traction beyond this context given that the symbolic meaning—of urban trash—communicated the controlling image of people who use drugs.

Such an association was used as justification for disproportionate arrest and incarceration of poor and then nonwhite populations. Although legislation made no explicit mention of race, in practice, communities were treated inequitably. The Harrison Narcotics Act of 1914—the nation's first foray into national drug legislation—rendered the recreational use of opium, morphine, cocaine, and heroin illegal while continuing to allow doctors to use and prescribe these substances as they deemed fit. Thus, these substances were transformed from remedies to poisons, but only when being used without the oversight of a doctor or the legal permission of the state. In other words, those with access to institutional permission slips, in the form of doctors' notes, were protected from this legislation.

Contemporary criminal approaches to substance use draw upon both the "junkie" and "Negro dope fiend" with their discussion of the "drugs lifestyle."[65] This term is commonly used among social workers and case managers to "refer to the perceived totalizing impacts of substance use." According to these practitioners, those embroiled in the "drugs lifestyle" are unable to delay gratification, tempted by things like sex or drugs, which distract attention from a normative work ethic.[66] Similar to Oscar Lewis's theory of a "culture of poverty" that sought to biologize both poverty and race,[67] the "drugs lifestyle" rhetoric offers a similarly totalizing identity that draws heavily upon racial, non-Western stereotypes of the uncivilized, nonwhite *other*. These were the very controlling images used to justify the enslavement of Black people on the grounds that they were feeble minded, lacked impulse control, and embodied brute strength, thereby necessitating supervision and protection by the white man.[68]

Despite that fact that the majority of those who use or sell substances illegally are white,[69] such racially motivated legislation fuels the misconception that low-income men of color use or sell mind-altering substances more frequently than white, affluent men or women. These controlling images are used to justify inequities in policing, arrests, and sentencing as it was *expected* that these groups would be overrepresented in the carceral system (it was the intention all along). This racial fallacy was exacerbated by the Comprehensive Drug Abuse Prevention and Control Act of 1969. The act classified narcotic and psychotropic drugs into five Schedules, based upon their alleged abuse potential, medical value, and safety—a schematic that coincidentally classified substances commonly used by white people as less harmful than substances used by nonwhite people. Schedule I drugs, deemed to be the most harmful, included heroin, marijuana, lysergic acid diethylamide (LSD), peyotes, and other hallucinogens. Substances classified as Schedule I were argued to have no medical or therapeutic use and therefore ought to be criminalized and punished with greatest severity by the criminal legal system. Morphine, opium, and codeine, as well as OxyContin, Percocet, and Dilaudid, were all considered to be Schedule II. Schedule II–V substances are considered to have some therapeutic value, depending on the context. This act enabled the systematic criminalization of substance use when not prescribed by a doctor while simultaneously facilitating legal discrimination against people who used certain categories of drugs. Users of Schedule II substances faced less severe penalties than those of Schedule I substances; however, without a doctor's oversight, an individual of either class faced penalty by the law.

Although the act was ostensibly introduced as a means of classifying substances in terms of harm, in practice, it resulted in the protection of certain classes of people (white and affluent) and punishment of others (nonwhite and poor) for the same behaviors.[70] This was made evident by the fact that alcohol and tobacco are conspicuously absent from the list of controlled substances. Despite the fact that alcohol causes greater harm than any other substance and cigarette smoke has been linked to lung cancer, high blood pressure, and other harmful or fatal conditions,[71] deaths by alcohol or tobacco use have different temporal horizons, as they take longer to produce fatal harms and their linkage to diseases is often indirect. Most importantly, they are not as closely associated with racial or class outgroups as substances such as crack cocaine, opium, or marijuana.

Richard Nixon signed the Comprehensive Drug Abuse Prevention and Control Act of 1969 into law, spurring a series of legislation that contributed to what legal scholar Michelle Alexander termed the "New Jim Crow."[72] Despite the fact that few Americans believed drug use to be a pressing national issue at the time (between 2 and 6 percent of those polled)[73] and that serving time in prison is associated with much greater harm than substance use itself, the act was passed under the guise of protecting drug users from harming themselves or others. However, the legislation was really about controlling "the antiwar left and black people," the "two enemies" of the Nixon administration. As the domestic policy adviser to President Nixon later admitted, "We knew we couldn't make it illegal to be either against the war or black, but by getting the public to associate the hippies with marijuana and blacks with heroin, and then criminalizing both heavily, we could disrupt those communities. We could arrest their leaders, raid their homes, break up their meetings, and vilify them night after night on the evening news. Did we know we were lying about the drugs? Of course we did."[74] In other words, the War on Drugs aimed to protect institutionalized racism and the inequalities that it produced, not the individuals using substances.

As part of the War on Drugs, the Justice Department made significant budgetary cuts to departments that interrogated and prosecuted white-collar crime and reassigned these personnel to focus on street crime, in particular, to drug-law enforcement.[75] This is notable because the very same departments that had their budgets cut in the 1970s were the ones responsible for investigating corporate fraud and malfeasance such as that which was happening at Purdue Pharma and other large companies engaged in wholesale fraud by misrepresenting the dangers posed by OxyContin and other opioids. The money was directed toward the Central Intelligence Agency, the Federal Bureau of Investigation, the Drug Enforcement Administration, and street crime units. While Jimmy Carter spent an average of $437 million a year on drug eradication between 1976 and 1980, Reagan spent on average $1.4 billion the following four years. During that same time, funding for substance use education, prevention, and rehabilitation was cut by $24 million.[76]

These changes to budgets, policies, and practices laid the groundwork for the development and proliferation of drug courts at the turn of the century, which effectively merged the field of medicine (by way of rehabilitation and treatment) with the carceral state. While introduced as a more humane, "therapeutic" alternative, in practice, it broadened the ability of both institutions to control and punish and stratified that punishment along lines of race, class, and gender. Further, by casting those who used certain substances as "bad actors" from whom the general public needed protection, the issue was individualized, requiring treatment or punishment on the individual level rather than structural reform.

Therapeutic Jurisprudence: Criminalizing the Victim,
Medicalizing the Criminal

On its face, it appears that addiction has been successfully medicalized given that it has shifted from an act of deviance to be dealt with by the criminal justice system to a medical problem to be treated by doctors and psychologists. However, treatment rarely comes from the medical profession. Instead, it is most often administered by people without medical training in rehabilitation programs that are required conditions of parole, probation, or drug court sentencing.[77] As a result, substance use, addiction, and treatment remain intimately linked with the carceral system and continue to be viewed through a moral lens.

The boundary between moral and immoral substance use is fundamental to legitimizing some groups and actions and delegitimizing others. While the criminal legal system has always been a mechanism for enforcement and punishment, the justification for such treatment has historically been religious. However, in the last century, medicine and science have usurped the role of defining and distinguishing between the healthy (moral, upstanding) and unhealthy (immoral, criminal).[78] While the medical use of prescription drugs is viewed as promoting moral, healthy, and productive labor, the nonmedical use of prescription drugs or illicit substances is viewed as interfering with and threatening both personal and community health, morality, and productivity. The boundary allows medical use—as defined and controlled by doctors and scientists—to remain legitimate, while use for pleasure is deemed illegitimate and destructive.

The medicalization of substance use is arguably more destructive than its earlier moralization given that an individual can repent for their sins and change their behavior. In contrast, a "chronic relapsing, brain disorder"[79] is a permanent diagnosis that warrants perpetual surveillance and control by both medical and criminal authorities given that use of illicit substances is simultaneously medicalized and criminalized. This is accomplished institutionally via the drug court system.

First introduced in Florida in 1989, drug courts deal with offenders who have been arrested by police on low-level, drug-related charges. Drug courts require an admission of guilt, a formal guilty plea, and compliance with a mandated treatment program in order to have clearance of criminal charges. Individuals are mandated to "volunteer" or partake in supervision for between one and two years, during which they frequently must attend an inpatient treatment, to be followed by randomized urine testing, group therapy, and obligatory sobriety meetings.[80]

These new programs reflect a "therapeutic" turn in prisons, where the criminal legal system seeks to reform rather than punish. As Foucault describes in *Discipline and Punish*, the focus of scrutiny shifts from the body—the object of corporal punishment—to the mind or the soul. On the surface, this shift sounds more humanistic, as it eliminates corporal punishment and violence. However, therapeutic jurisprudence suggests this shift has become more punitive and coercive than prior models. Therapeutic jurisprudence locates criminal offending within the psyches of the offenders. As a consequence, treatment involves reshaping the brain, breaking down individuals in order to build them back up in the image of the "good citizen" as defined by those designing and implementing the programs. In her ethnographic study of a women's rehabilitation center, sociologist Jill McCorkel describes how these programs assume that the person is incapable of self-regulation and therefore needs to be supervised by external forces. Addiction could be understood as "a disorder of the whole person. The problem is the person, not the drug."[81] Accordingly, "it is a self that must be surrendered to a lifelong process of external management and control."[82] There is no escape from the carceral system in such a model, whose cure is only more treatment or punishment.

This is particularly acute for the already marginalized, given that treatment is stratified by race and class. While "whiter and richer drug offenders are filtered out to non-custodial community care," the nonwhite, poorer, "'criminal addict' is held to strict accountability within the quasi-incarceration of the strongarm rehab."[83] This "therapeutic" approach reflects a paternalistic one that presents itself benevolently via psychiatric professions that require individuals to remake their identities so as to conform to prototypical images of the good citizen: sober, gainfully employed, and supporting a family.

As sociologist Kerwin Kaye argues, drug courts and therapeutic communities are often appealing to both law-and-order conservatives and reformist liberals as they promise "accountability and cost savings" while also offering "an alternative to mass incarceration that addresses the root causes of drug use and criminality in a more humane manner."[84] What many do not realize is that this "alternative" only extends the punishment, as individuals must plead guilty to full charges—associated with harshest penalties—to enter such programs. Although they are spared these penalties if they follow the conditions of "treatment," if they fail on account of being caught with drugs in their system or violating conditions of probation, they are immediately sentenced to the fullest extent of the law. These sentences are often much more severe than if they had been able to enter into a plea bargain or been able to successfully defend their innocence in the first place. As a consequence, drug courts extend and intensify punishment both in terms of traditional carceral punishment and in terms of the "adoption of a disease model of addiction [that] thereby seeks to justify the court's existence in retributive terms as well as rehabilitative, enabling it to speak to diverse audiences in different contexts."[85]

The threat of imprisonment looms large during the entire drug court process, given that drug use itself is a crime. Therefore, relapse means recidivism. Those sentenced to detox and treatment as part of the drug court system "are dually and contradictorily marked; the addict/offender is both patient and prisoner."[86] Such a dual construction sets up the patient-prisoner to be diagnosed, treated, and rehabilitated by the dual forces of medical and carceral power as they are shuffled between institutions and overseen by different doctors, wardens, and counselors.

Reliance upon pharmacological solutions coupled with the erection of a medical-penal structure to regulate, treat, and punish substance use produces what I have termed a prescription-to-prison pipeline. This builds upon the scholarship outlined above that has chronicled (1) how endemic social problems have been biologized, externalized, or criminalized, (2) how the so-called therapeutic turn has further entrenched and intensified the punishment process, and (3) how existing inequalities are often only further exacerbated by medicalization and criminalization processes.[87] The prescription-to-prison pipeline is the pharmaco-socio-political structure that results in the treatment of social issues such as poverty, trauma, abuse, and racism as biomedical, presenting opioid or psychotropic substances as solutions to those problems while subsequently surveilling and punishing certain groups or individuals for engaging in these practices without institutional consent. It refers to the discursive, neoliberal pressures upon individuals who have not been prescribed medication to seek out ways to self-medicate as well as those who have been prescribed medication by doctors but who then adapt treatment based on their embodied experiences. Without broader social support or sufficient health-care support, prescription medications are often perceived as a legitimate source of support as they are produced in well-funded laboratories, marketed by profitable pharmaceutical companies, and prescribed by benevolent doctors. However, for those subjected to greater carceral surveillance as a consequence of their race, class, gender, social location, or interaction with institutions of control (e.g., foster care, prison), use of prescription medication can quickly be transformed into abuse, thereby closing rather than opening doors.

The remainder of this book chronicles the stories of those who became ensnared in the prescription-to-prison pipeline by virtue of different life experiences that intensified pain or exposed them to greater state surveillance. Stories sometimes begin with pain that was managed through prescription and later classified as abuse, resulting in criminalization and incarceration. However, other stories begin without pain. In these accounts, behaviors of certain populations are deemed problematic by institutional authorities and thereby in need of either pharmacological or carceral intervention. While these processes begin in different places through different processes, the result is the same—a pipeline into medical and legal systems that define such behavior through a lens of chronicity, thereby warranting perpetual surveillance and control. In expecting recidivism and relapse, regular contact with agents of power and institutional interventions become the norm, as do their associated harms. Separating these stories into stages of the prescription-to-prison pipeline, while difficult, helps demonstrate how the pipeline operates.

PRESCRIPTION

GETTING HOOKED

Penny, a thirty-nine-year-old white woman, grew up in a tumultuous house-hold where her father, who was "an alcoholic and a drug addict," would physi-cally abuse her mother, and her "mom would beat [Penny] up when she'd get stressed out." In response to physical injuries and psychological trauma, Penny had been prescribed "Percocet . . . Xanax . . . Darvocet . . . Vicodin. Just about every pill. Every pain pill, I had." From a young age, Penny had learned to medi-cate both physical and psychological violence with prescription drugs. She had used them on and off for over a decade.

Then, when she gave birth, Penny was prescribed more pain pills following a cesarean section. She was prescribed both Percocet and Xanax for six months and Penny used up every one. When the scripts finally ran out, Penny went through intense withdrawal. She was home with a newborn and her body was depleted. She started to spiral as she struggled to care for her daughter while her vision was blurred, her body shook uncontrollably, and her mind raced with frantic and anxious thoughts. She didn't know where to turn or what to do, so she did what she thought it would take to get doctors to refill her scripts—she proved that she needed them. She created pain that they would see as legitimate and warranting medication. Penny describes how she "had someone hit [her] with a baseball bat," so she could get more pills. She recalls,

> I've jumped out of trees, I've done all kinds of stuff. Banged my hand on a wall until it swelled up so big that it obviously was painful. I cut my finger open all the way to the bone, my whole finger—I would have done anything short of cutting my own limb off, I would have. I can't say that there would never have been a point where it got to that. And then I'd get infections; my finger got infected, after I cut it open. And I wouldn't go to the doctor. Well, I would go to the doctor, but I wouldn't take the antibiotics, so that it would stay bad.

Penny explains she would use these medications for "everything: depression, PTSD, just, you know, life in general."

Penny's doctor shopping—the practice of obtaining prescriptions from different doctors or filling them at multiple pharmacies to maximize the amount of acquired medication—eventually resulted in arrest and imprisonment. At the time of her interview, she was in prison on charges of domestic violence, forgery, and tampering with a motor vehicle, all while under the influence of Vicodin. Penny, like many others, was initially prescribed medication to manage her anxiety, to help her recover from childbirth, to manage postpartum depression and anxiety, and to help her stay focused at work. But her scripts lasted only so long. When they ran out, Penny would do anything to get more.

Prescription drug use has become so normalized in the United States that it has become routine practice to use them even in the absence of symptoms. Despite the fact that the vast majority of Americans rate their health as excellent (35.9 percent), very good (30.1 percent), or good (23.9 percent), as of 2012, half of all US adults were diagnosed as "suffering" from at least one "chronic disease."[1] This language paints a dire picture that directly contradicts other measures of health, such as life expectancy, which is considerably longer today than in centuries past. These data reveal how prescription drugs have been reconceptualized from a cure for a specific disease to a means of maintaining health and preventing risk.

Between 2015 and 2018, 10 percent of the US population had used an opioid in any given thirty-day period.[2] Given the ubiquity of these medications, and because they had been prescribed directly from a doctor, many interviewees thought that prescription drugs were benign. Gina didn't consider pills dangerous because "I wasn't on the street getting it. I was getting it from a reputable doctor with my name on the prescription." Similarly, Lyndsey argued, "My doctor gave them to me, therefore it can't be that bad." Gina is a Black woman with a master's degree; Lyndsey, a white woman who never completed high school. And yet they both felt some level of trust for medical professionals. People often explained that they used prescription drugs because a doctor had prescribed them and therefore they felt more "healthy" or "respectable" than street drugs. It never crossed their minds that prescription drug use might eventually result in their incarceration.

As Rhianna, a twenty-five-year-old white woman, summarized, "When you think of pills, everybody uses pills, doctors prescribe you pills. It's got a better reputation. Everybody uses pills." It is true that the majority of Americans use prescription medication. And yet, what type of medication is prescribed and how that medication is treated by medical and legal systems vary by gender, race, and class.

In this chapter, I explore how and why interviewees initially started using prescription drugs—stories that often began in a doctor's office. I explore how everyday events have become increasingly medicalized. I draw attention to the reverberating effects that are produced when previously nonmedical events become medicalized.

Prescription drugs are increasingly offered as an individualized solution to collective social problems. This reflects an American bootstrap worldview that assumes individuals are personally responsible for pulling themselves out of structural inequality and marginalization. In this chapter, I highlight different avenues by which individuals began using prescription drugs. While these are often presented in individualist, corporeal terms (injury, surgery, childbirth, abuse), the pain is often the result of the same neoliberal capitalist society that promotes individual-level solutions.

"A Capable Employee, but with a Habit": Work and Prescription Drugs

Ronald was a fifty-three-year-old white man who worked in construction. He describes how he regularly worked "twelve- to fourteen-hour shifts lifting five-eighths-inch-thick, twelve-foot-long by four-foot-wide sheets of Sheetrock all day long. It's an amazingly hard job. It's like three hundred pounds apiece, and I had to do it by myself." He would routinely come home from work physically exhausted, go to bed early, and wake up sore and in pain. Several times, he had materials such as Sheetrock or metal beams drop on him at work. These incidents resulted in head trauma and concussions. While he was given time off, he never complained about lingering symptoms, such as migraines and blurred vision, for fear of losing his job. With only a high school diploma, Ron felt that his job prospects were limited to manual labor. At a time when he feared he might not have the physical strength left to continue in his line of work, he started dating a woman who suggested he try "Ritalin, or the Adderalls." While he was initially reticent, having never taken any substances other than alcohol before, during a particularly grueling job, he decided to try them out. It was like night and day. He recalled, "I'd take one, break it in half, and it'd get me through a twelve- to sixteen-hour shift at work." From his perspective, "the Adderall were really a necessary component . . . the job was beyond my physical capability, so I medicated to be able to perform." Ron took Ritalin and Adderall for years before another friend suggested methamphetamines to give him an extra boost of energy. His methamphetamine use resulted in incarceration.

Low-wage jobs often result in pain. There are many risk factors to such work, including physically strenuous labor, inflexible schedules, lack of paid sick leave or health insurance, and the need to work long hours (and often multiple jobs) to cover basic living expenses. Together, these factors increase the likelihood for negative health outcomes. Given that low-wage jobs often require workers to be physically present and mobile during their shifts, workers have less time to cook home-prepared meals, to exercise, to take vitamins or medications, to see doctors, or to engage in other preventive care. As a consequence, they are more likely to suffer from poor nutrition and poor health and to be vulnerable to injury and disease.

Such was the case for Aiden, a fifty-three-year-old white man, who had "had back problems ever since [he] was twenty years old." Aiden had also worked for most of his life in construction and had been in a number of car accidents while on the job. After one work injury, Aiden went to a doctor who prescribed him Vicodin, and it helped manage the pain. While it had been helpful, he never went back to the doctor because he didn't have health insurance and didn't realize how much that doctor's visit would cost him. Aiden worked "in asphalt for the last twenty years, and it's hot and it's hard work. I don't know, if you've had a long day . . . the next morning comes around pretty quick." Still in pain, Aiden complained to friends, who quickly suggested he split their prescriptions or recommended others who would sell prescriptions that had been covered by their insurance for extra cash. Aiden took them up on their offers. As he described it, "I would take a couple Vicodin and it speed me." Vicodin simultaneously masked his pain and gave him the energy to manage long work hours—as he describes, "speeding" his actions. Enjoying these effects, Aiden started using Vicodin regularly "just to stay working . . . to stay medicated to stay working." Those with access to health care are prescribed drugs to manage work injuries or chronic pain; however, those who cannot afford to see a doctor may learn about prescription drugs from coworkers, family, or friends who suffered from the same pains and have found nonmedical ways of coping.

Of the fifty richest nations in the world, the United States is the only country that does not provide universal health-care coverage to its citizens.[3] As a result, Americans must obtain health coverage through their employers, through Medicaid (for those who qualify based on income) or Medicare (for those over sixty-five years of age),[4] or by purchasing it on a free market. Prior to implementation of the Affordable Care Act in 2010, 48.6 million Americans (16 percent) were not covered by health insurance at all.[5] Some could not afford coverage, while others were denied coverage by insurance companies because they had preexisting medical conditions that cost more to cover and treat and therefore were not profitable for health insurance to cover. Even after the implementation of the Affordable Care Act, twenty-six million Americans remain uninsured—mostly in states that refused to expand Medicaid coverage to assist those who cannot afford to pay for coverage, or that have added work requirements to qualify for benefits.[6] Missouri, the site of this study, is one of the states with the most restrictive requirements for Medicaid eligibility, and the Republican governor, Mike Parsons, denied coverage to eligible low-income adults even after such expansion had been approved by a state-wide popular vote in 2020.

Low-wage jobs rarely provide health insurance or paid time off for their employees. This is especially true for the very jobs where one is most likely to become injured or develop chronic pain, such as construction work, manual labor, or jobs that involve repetitive motions or standing or sitting without reprieve. If an employee does become sick or injured, they risk losing their job, so many interviewees took their health into their own hands, self-medicating injuries and seeking out alternative ways to support their families. Pauline, a thirty-two-year-old white woman with a high school diploma, argued that prescription drugs "made me a harder worker, I was able to get more done, I was more focused when I was using." Stacey, a thirty-two-year-old white woman with some college education, argued that the prescription drugs "made me a capable employee, but with a habit."

In fact, some employers played a role in this process, going so far as to medicate employees on the job site to keep them from taking time off. Rachel, a twenty-seven-year-old white woman with some college education, describes how she was prescribed Percocet from a doctor at her workplace: "I used to work at this factory. I worked the floor, twelve hours a day, seven days a week. My legs and stuff would hurt a lot." She explains how "you can get prescribed pills for working in them factories, because they know you're standing on your feet every day. They prescribe you if it makes you be a better worker, but if you're taking above what you're supposed to take, which most people end up having to anyways, it can mess you up at work." In Rachel's case, her employer recognized that it was not sustainable to require employees to work twelve-hour shifts on their feet for seven days per week. Employees were too tired and too prone to injury. However, instead of reducing hours and paying workers more, the employer decided that the solution was to medicate the injuries and medicate the exhaustion. Rather than restructure the environment that produces these harms, the solution is simple: take a pill.

The experience of feeling poor in a society of plenty, specifically in a meritocratic society in which people are blamed for being poor, has an intense negative effect on one's health.[7] The prospect of working low-wage jobs can impel some to get involved in the street drug market while others might self-medicate due to depression or feelings of inferiority. Such was the case for Walter, a sixty-five-year-old Black man, who started using prescription drugs after a medical leave forced him to abandon his education, which he perceived as his only opportunity for upward class mobility. Walter was doing it all. He "was landscaping, home remodeling and landscaping, and going to school" for "computer programming" at night. It was challenging juggling work and school, but it gave him hope for a better job that would be easier on his aging body. He was a semester away from completing his degree, but then he "started losing [his] sight." Unbeknownst to him, Walter was born with a degenerative eye disorder that manifested in midlife. Learning of his diagnosis was crushing. He remembers, "[I] had a goal and I had accomplished a goal short range and I was building life from this here step by step on the way out the door I had planned and planned and planned. And I worked hard for three or four years in a row and it was going to manifest itself. . . . I had a life to look forward to." But then he lost his vision and he describes how "I had to take a medical leave. And I couldn't finish it and then it caused me to be depressed as hell, caused me to be angry 'cause I'd worked so hard to do it."

Walter describes getting so close to his goal only to have it taken away from him: it "made me bitter and it made me . . . I knew what I had to give up and I couldn't do nothing about my sight. I had to be patient and I didn't want to be patient and then that pissed me off even more." Walter ended up taking a leave of absence, but when he realized his vision would never return, his occupational aspirations felt out of reach. He was initially prescribed medication for his physical symptoms of the degenerative disorder, but Water continued taking it longer to manage emotional pain and "to keep from using those other drugs" such as heroin or meth. More than anything, Walter did not want to be a patient or a victim. He wanted to take control of his own life—supporting himself and his family. He wanted to take his future into his own hands, but during the course of his struggles, he became a prisoner instead.

Increasingly, the labor market is divided between (1) those who do mental labor, who can work from home on their own schedules and get paid enough to afford leisure time during which they can exercise or cook fresh food, and (2) those who do physical labor, who must be physically present and active at work, are confined to rigid schedules, and are paid insufficiently to be able to afford healthy food, health care, or time to unwind. The cruel irony is that those in the former category are more likely to be insured and able to attend doctor's appointments with secure and reliable transportation, whereas those engaged in low-wage labor are less likely to be insured, less likely to have reliable transportation, and less likely to have the ability to take time off from work to receive care.[8] As a result, the options for pain management are stratified by class and occupation, as well as gender.

"I Felt like Super Mom When I Was on Them": Motherhood and Prescription Drugs

Alone in a gas station bathroom, Katie peed on a stick. There were two pink lines. It couldn't be right. But she bought another and the result was the same. She had put on weight recently but couldn't figure out why. Now she knew. She was fourteen years old and pregnant. When she told her mom, she was kicked out of the house. Without health insurance or the ability to support herself, Katie dropped out of high school. She moved in with her boyfriend—who was several years older and had a place of his own—but that was short-lived as he became physically and emotionally abusive, and Katie feared for her life.

While she hadn't had access to birth control or reproductive care before or during her pregnancy, once she was in the hospital giving birth, Katie was offered a panoply of medical care, including prescription drugs. During labor, her baby's heartbeat slowed so Katie was given an emergency cesarean section that did not heal as it should have. She was prescribed Percocet for her recovery. Afterward, the doctors generously filled and refilled her prescriptions, and as Katie describes, "that was it, for five years, I was straight addicted to opiates, bad. Wasn't getting up, wasn't cooking dinner, you know, my paychecks go to it, not going to work unless I have it." At seventeen, Katie was living on her own, supporting herself and her child, all while trying to finish school. Without financial or social support, she turned to the one form of support she did have: prescription drugs.

The medicalization of childbirth reflects how social, economic, and political issues such as gender inequality in the home, at work, and in politics have been turned into biological issues to be remedied with medication. This was true for Katie, who used prescription drugs to recover from surgery but also to "self-medicate" for other pains, including poverty, depression, unresolved childhood trauma, and isolation as a low-income single mother. She describes how opiates gave her the energy to manage her responsibilities as a mother; "especially just after having a baby, you know, it takes away that baby blues and gives you energy."

Marginalized mothers, by virtue of their class or race, are often evaluated against white, upper-middle-class norms of motherhood, even when they lack the resources requisite to adhere to them.[9] This reflects neoliberal pressures upon motherhood, whereby individuals—rather than communities—are responsible for providing financial, emotional, and social resources for children and mothers. Prescription drugs offer a means to amplify one's abilities in the absence of other such resources. Prescription drugs have a long history of being prescribed to white, middle-class mothers in order to manage so-called healthy levels of emotionality and to follow norms of "good mothering." Such medication regimes promote a chemical treatment for postpartum depression, anxiety, stress, and body maintenance rather than calling into question the systems that produce and exacerbate these ailments.[10] Instead of focusing on the absence of parental leave policies, the unaffordability of childcare, or the incompatibility between traditional working hours and grade school hours, our society considers women who express discomfort or stress with balancing competing demands to be biologically and emotionally unstable. Rather than changing the underlying social structures that produce undue financial, emotional, and social stress on caretakers, the preferred solution is medication, which imperfectly addresses the inevitable symptoms of such an environment. Such medicalization of motherhood in the absence of a corresponding medicalization of fatherhood illustrates this gender disparity and how medicine exacerbates, rather than ameliorates, gender inequities. This divergence begins for many women during pregnancy and childbirth.

The practice of prescribing pain pills to new mothers has increasingly become the norm in the United States as childbirth has become a medicalized event. Over 99 percent of births in the United States take place in hospitals, and as of 2013, over one-third of those ended in a cesarean section (C-section), more than double the rate of 10–15 percent that the World Health Organization

(WHO) recommends.[11] The WHO's recommended rate reflects the fact that C-section deliveries are associated with more frequent occurrences of injury and death for both mother and child than occur with vaginal birth deliveries,[12] and they were designed to be used only in emergency or unique circumstances. While C-sections can be lifesaving operations, the C-section is also a serious surgical procedure that often requires weeks of recovery—and narcotics to manage pain.

Paralleling national trends, over a third of the women interviewed for this book had been prescribed pain pills after a cesarean section.[13] Lauren, a thirty-year-old white woman, was one of the women who began using prescription drugs after a cesarean childbirth. She describes how she "had a C-section that they screwed up pretty bad" and, as a result, was prescribed OxyContin and Percocet. Prescription drugs "helped [her] after the surgeries to be able to get around." Her prescriptions helped her both physically and emotionally. She describes how she "felt like super mom when I was on them because I could get everything done that I needed to, and not have the postpartum blues about not doing this or that. It just made me forget about problems." Recovering from a C-section takes considerable time, and women who feel the pressures to take care of their children and their homes, as well as maintain paid labor, are often faced with an untenable situation. The prescription drugs offer one way of medicating physical pain and managing intense postpartum emotions.

Cesarean sections can result in negative future reproductive consequences for the mother, increase the recovery time for mothers after giving birth, and cost almost twice as much as vaginal deliveries. While physicians and pregnant women are often blamed for the soaring rise of C-section rates, sociologist Theresa Morris argues that the spike in cesarean sections in the United States can be attributed to economic, legal, and political structures. Despite unfounded claims that "older women, larger women, women who gain excess weight in pregnancy, women of color, and women with private insurance" or women who are "too posh to push" are more likely to have a C-section, the rate of C-sections has gone up among *all* women in the last thirty years.[14] Morris attributes the rise in C-section rates to increases in both the malpractice insurance market and the size of medical practices, resulting in a hyperstandardization of care that limits the autonomy of health-care providers on the pretext of protecting them from liability.[15]

Despite the fact that most women and maternity providers claim they do not prefer C-sections over vaginal births (which do not require surgical intervention), the choices of both women and maternity providers are limited by organizational constraints, such as reprimand from a supervisor, poor rating, or the denial of coverage by insurance companies and Medicaid.[16] The impact of organizational constraints can have dire consequences for individuals who give birth.

Mothering at the margins involves extensive efforts, and many women described how Rx drugs helped them fulfill key obligations to dependents by helping them "cope" or "hold [themselves] together" as well as "keeping the family together." The identity of being a good mother was a central theme that appeared in all the interviews with mothers, as well as with two others who wished that they had become mothers. Of the thirty-four women in the interview sample who had children, twenty-six (76 percent) were single mothers at some point while raising their children, making daily responsibilities even more burdensome. For example, Rhianna argued that Klonopin and Adderall helped her with pleasing her partner "sexually, cleaning the house, taking care of things. . . . [They] would get you going. I was wonder woman. Especially after having kids. . . . I think it helped me keep my house clean and keep my cool. The food we did have, I didn't have to eat as much of. I had the energy to deal with my kids." For Rhianna, prescription drugs helped her with childcare, housework, and dieting, as well as sexual relations with her partner.

Betsy, a thirty-three-year-old white woman who dropped out of high school, describes how oxycodone "helped with [her] pain": "I was able to do things that usually I couldn't do, chase after my kid. Usually, I'm just like, Let her go. I ain't got it, I ain't got it in me to get her. I just don't. . . . I'd hang onto her because I could not run after her because I was in pain. When I took oxycodone, I could run after her. I could keep up with her all day long."

Nancy, another thirty-three-year-old white woman, described how opioids gave her "an amazing euphoric high. You can just take on the world and everything was happy-go-lucky. Oh, you could spot-clean your house and sit down and still have energy to help your kid with the homework. Yeah, then I figured I'd be smart to use it as just a motivational drug." Women explained how prescription drugs helped them fulfill the competing responsibilities of womanhood, motherhood, and being a breadwinner—caretaking, homemaking, working, and controlling the body. Instead of structural reform at the political, social, or economic level, the medicalization of these ailments and struggles offered an individual-level solution: prescription drugs.

The impacts of medicalization and pharmaceuticalization extend beyond the childbirth process; many women described how they used prescription drugs in order to "do it all." As such pharmacological interventions were encouraged during both pregnancy and childbirth, once mothers left the hospital, they often described feeling overwhelmed and unable to meet the competing demands of breadwinning and childrearing in the absence of structural or social support; a pharmacological solution wasn't enough. In her research, sociologist Caitlin Collins argues that such inequalities are the result not only of inadequate work-family policies but also of enduring cultural beliefs about gender inequality, employment, and motherhood that put pressure upon mothers—rather than fathers—to take on the majority of caretaking work, even when they must also work full time.[17]

As many as one in five mothers experiences postpartum depression or anxiety. In order to help identify and treat these conditions, doctors who see mothers, as well as pediatricians who see newborns with their mothers, engage in formal assessments of mothers' postpartum psychological condition at each appointment. While these practices help identify these conditions, oftentimes the treatment prescribed to those who are diagnosed is exclusively pharmacological rather than social, financial, or psychological. This appears to be true for many of the mothers whom we spoke to. For example, Tonya, a forty-nine-year-old white woman with a high school education, describes, "I honestly thought, 'Nobody knows that I'm taking what I'm taking, I'm a good mom, I'm a good wife. I can do anything I want. Nobody is gonna know.'" Further, Tonya felt as though these substances helped her emulate the ideal. She describes how, when she was on pills, "[I'd] get up, I'd be happy, I'd go through the day doing all kinds of stuff, just as nice as it could be. When I ran out of pills or it started to get to the point where I needed more, I'd be kind of crappy and just nasty and . . . but I thought, 'Oh a lot of time I take these [and] I feel a lot better and, you know, I'm a nicer person so I'm gonna keep doing it.'" Tonya describes how while using them she felt "completely alone" so she decided to just "keep self-medicating." But then, "it just got worse and worse because I just, 'OK, well, nobody cares so I'm just gonna take more and more pills.'" Raising children on her own without steady employment or safe and affordable housing, Tonya felt overwhelmed and fearful. "Self-medicating" with the drugs that she had initially been prescribed for postpartum depression was her primary coping mechanism, until it landed her in prison. Tonya was arrested and charged with writing a fake check in order to buy more prescription drugs.

"Numbing Myself from the Pain": Trauma and Prescription Drugs

"We ran down a trail, you know. I never saw him coming. He drug me down into a drainage ditch and raped me. It was horrible. . . . I was nineteen. And when I tell you I was done, I was *done*." Francis's story—a stranger jumping out of the woods and violently raping her—reflects a dominant cultural prototype of rape. However, most sexual assaults do not resemble this trope. A stranger in the woods is much less likely to be one's assailant than one's parent, intimate partner, or close friend. By narrowing cultural focus to the random violent stranger, other, more prevalent, forms of sexual assault are often neglected, such as the many experiences of sexual abuse that Francis—a thirty-nine-year-old white woman—experienced before this final harrowing assault.

Long before she was attacked in the woods, Francis was molested by her mother as a child. She didn't label these experiences as molestation until much later in her life when she was confronted by a therapist. When she was twelve, Francis was raped by a friend's twenty-year-old brother, while her friend was raped by her brother's friend. The two twelve-year-old girls never reported the incident; instead, "[we] made this little pact that we were never going to tell, we were just going to get them back someday, we thought." Francis managed to keep these traumas to herself, bottling up her anger and fear over the years. But then when she was raped by a stranger, as recounted above, she finally broke down. Francis believed that this experience hit her harder than previous experiences, in part because after raping her, the stranger "left [her] for dead."

Francis was found by a passerby who reported the situation to the police, which forced Francis to identify and label the experience as rape. This may also have been consequential given that the majority of sexual assault survivors do not identify their attack as "rape" out of shame or self-preservation and often do not report violations to authorities. Survivors fear the repercussions on social ties—being excommunicated from the family or admonished by a group of friends. In work or school settings, survivors fear reporting given how it might impact their education or career paths. Accusations can threaten job security, not just of the assailant but also of the survivor, who could be accused of falsely "crying rape"—an expression that itself cements a false cultural myth.[18]

Despite the fact that one in five women will experience some form of sexual violence in their lifetime and close to half of those who identify as LGBTQ are also survivors of sexual assault, only a quarter of those report those assaults to authorities.[19] While false accusations of sexual assault are exceedingly rare— no different from the rate of false accusations of burglary, arson, homicide, or other violent acts—the myth that rape is something often falsely reported scares many into silence, seeing nothing to be gained from a system that is more likely to end in gaslighting or shame than in justice.[20]

Sexual assault is an act of violence in and of itself, but the very threat of it produces and reproduces "gendered dominance in everyday interaction,"[21] which influences one's behavior and one's self-concept. Given pervasive myths that individuals "did something" to be assaulted, many survivors blame themselves rather than the perpetrators or the institutions and cultures that allow the perpetrators to evade accountability and remediation.

Three-quarters of the women (thirty out of forty) interviewed for this book had been sexually abused, a finding that parallels other samples of incarcerated women.[22] Many of them kept these experiences to themselves because they felt responsible or because they feared that the consequences might only exacerbate their problems. As a result, many abuses go unreported, and survivors find their own ways to cope. Many survivors are conflicted on whether they want their assailants to be punished if it may result in further community violence. For example, although Ingrid's adoptive father molested her as a child, she reflected, "I'm glad that he didn't go to jail because it would have really torn my mom up and done even more damage to our family." This desire to "keep the family together" began at a very young age, before Ingrid, a thirty-nine-year-old white woman with a high school diploma, herself was a mother. This speaks to the current family demographics of the most disadvantaged in America, who are disproportionately impacted by mass incarceration.

The experience of having one's assault denied or covered up by loved ones was not uncommon among interviewees and contributed to a sense of feeling unsafe or unprotected from an early age. For example, when Janice, a thirty-nine-year-old white woman with a high school diploma, was five years old, her father's "best friend, [whom] I considered my uncle, raped me." Her father knew about the sexual abuse and did nothing. Similarly, Whitney, a twenty-year-old white woman who dropped out of high school, describes the impacts of her mother staying together with her stepfather after he raped her when she was thirteen years old. Rather than press charges, Whitney's mother suggested that she see a psychiatrist, who prescribed Whitney Xanax. Instead of there being action taken that involved the perpetrator—her stepfather—Whitney was the one who had to manage the situation through medication. She described how she would "numb" herself from the pain. It is this self-medication that eventually resulted in arrest and imprisonment. When interviewed, she was incarcerated on charges of possession of opiates and hydrocodone.

While sexual abuse is more commonly experienced by girls, women, nonbinary, and trans people, experiences that are reported by boys and men are often disbelieved, compounding the trauma. For example, Paul, a fifty-five-year-old multiracial man, describes: "[I] was molested by my aunt. And that's traumatizing, even still today. And when I told Mom about it, she said, 'Naw, women don't do that.'" Paul's father drank a lot and was rarely home. His mother was his one source of support, and when she didn't believe him, he was crushed.

As a result, Paul "start[ed] withdrawing from people then. I just did my own little thing. I never talked to a lot of people, even my brothers and sisters. So, that's when I started my withdrawal stages. All I did was worry about school. So that's why I was a straight A student all the way until I was seventeen. [Then I] went into the military just to get away." Paul's survival strategy was to sever ties with his family and friends and try to create a new life. However, without a support network, he struggled. He saw a psychiatrist after his service and was prescribed a number of benzodiazepines and SSRIs to manage his depression and anxiety. Medication became the means of coping. It also became the reason for his incarceration. At the time of the interview, Paul was serving his fourth sentence in prison and had been arrested over fifty times. Paul's life struggles were both medicalized and criminalized, exacerbating the inequities produced by structural conditions.

"Three Kids All by Myself, No Job, No Ride, Living on $200 a Month": Pharmacological Solutions for Structural Problems

Alejandro, a fifty-three-year-old white and Native American man, grew up on the South Side of Chicago. His father was shot and killed by a police officer when Alejandro was ten years old. His mother had limited education and struggled to find work as she had been forced to drop out of school in the fourth grade to help take care of younger siblings. Without a high school diploma, supporting her children and herself proved challenging on her own. She managed to find employment, but it was often minimum-wage work that didn't cover the bills. For a couple of years, she was dating a man who moved in and helped pay the expenses, but the relationship quickly deteriorated when he began "to rob her every first of the month for her money, [while] he was on heroin." It was incredibly painful for Alejandro to watch his mother struggle to keep them afloat. From a young age, he desperately wanted to help out. Without her consent or knowledge, Alejandro started selling drugs. It brought him joy to be able to alleviate some of her stress and contribute to the family. When she asked where the money came from, he lied, saying he had started working at the corner store.

After a couple of years, Alejandro was arrested on drug charges and sent to a juvenile detention facility, where he was diagnosed with "ADHD type stuff, then it turned into Bipolar." Alejandro refers to being diagnosed with attention-deficit/hyperactivity disorder, which impacts one's ability to focus, as well as bipolar disorder, which significantly impacts one's mood. While in custody, Alejandro was prescribed a laundry list of medications: Ritalin for "mental issues," Seroquel and Quaalude for "sleeping," and Valium and Ativan for "anxiety." Alejandro's childhood was traumatic—losing a father to police violence, growing up in a neighborhood where he'd "see people dying, and they'd be laying in the like, doorway . . . [for] two or three days," and growing up so poor that neither food nor housing was a thing he could reliably expect. Instead of someone working with him to process and cope with these challenges, Alejandro's problems were treated as though they were the product of his biology rather than structural inequalities.

Alejandro is currently in prison on charges of a probation violation and driving with a revoked license. In other words, Alejandro is incarcerated as a result of the net-widening effects of the carceral system whereby probation, parole and its associated surveillance, and financial debt make it more likely that he will reoffend and end up back in prison. Those who have run-ins with the law at a young age are subjected to heightened surveillance and compounding punishment that only intensify the effects of the punitive system on children who were already less likely to have access to resources and support. Yet, the use of medical diagnoses and prescription drugs as an additional layer of surveillance and control is notable, given that these very substances were the grounds for subsequent arrest and incarceration.

Those who experience adversity as children are disproportionately more likely to be diagnosed with and medicated for a psychological disorder than those who do not. Several studies estimate that close to 100 percent of children who have experienced three or more adverse childhood events (ACE), such as violence, poverty, or neglect, are diagnosed with a psychological disorder later in life.[23] Of those, many go untreated or are undertreated, failing to receive adequate follow-up care or oversight to assure effective treatment. In fact, only four out of ten US adults with a mental health condition received mental health services in 2015, and only half of children with a mental health condition received care in that same year.[24] If they are treated at all, it is often through psychotropics.[25] This is problematic given that, on average, people who suffer from depression, post-traumatic stress disorder, or anxiety experience greater relief of symptoms from therapeutic treatments as compared to pharmacological ones. Such pharmacological modi operandi may also explain why children who experience emotional, physical, or psychological trauma are much more likely to use illicit drugs, given that they were taught to manage pain and the symptoms of trauma with pharmacological substances.[26]

Betsy, a thirty-three-year-old white woman who did not complete high school, tells a similar story. Raised in an abusive and unstable family, she was "put on Xanax when I was seventeen. This is where it started really, the pills. When I was seventeen years old I went in to see a psychiatrist and said, 'I'm having anxiety and I'm depressed.' I was on Medicaid. Bam, just like that, Xanax here you go, just wrote me a prescription. He didn't even listen to what I said, didn't care. He wrote me a prescription and sent me on my way with Xanax, five blues a day, 150 a month. He destroyed my life."

Years after her initial prescription of Xanax, Betsy was diagnosed with rheumatoid arthritis and was prescribed Percocet and other narcotics to manage the pain associated with both the disease and spousal abuse. She describes how "my husband beat me up every day for twelve years. Ran me over with the car, threw me down steps, kicked me in the stomach when I was pregnant with my daughter, Callie, and he would kick his baby with steel-toe boots on and stuff like that." In excruciating pain, Betsy went to a doctor for help. But without financial or social support to move out, she was stuck in the relationship and cycle of abuse. The doctor prescribed more medication.

At the time of her arrest, Betsy was living with her mother, her newborn, and her two other children in a "very high stress situation" given that Betsy's mother was "a paranoid schizophrenic" who had "been mentally ill [her] whole life." Betsy did not want to live with her mother, but she couldn't afford to live on her own. She describes how she "was under a lot of stress, a lot of pressure, three kids all by myself, no job, no ride, living on $200 a month." Under these conditions, Betsy started taking more of her prescribed medication than she had been prescribed. These included Percocet (an opioid painkiller), Xanax (a sedative), and Soma (muscle relaxants). While under the influence of these substances, she tried to give her infant son a bath. She nodded off, and he drowned. The medications were intended to help Betsy manage her psychological pain. They resulted in her imprisonment.

With pain in her voice, Betsy remarks, "I'm a baby killer and I'm no good. I was all over the news, and they splattered me and talked about all the Betsys in the world and how they live off the government and this, this, and that. Little do they know is that their government is what made me a junkie." Betsy describes how she was used as a political example of a bad mother who should not be eligible for government subsidies or support; however, her situation began as a result of inadequate health care and social and economic support. Chronically underemployed and unhoused, and with minimal childcare support, Betsy had few options as a single mother tasked with caring for her mother and three children. From her perspective, Betsy's outcomes were the result of a deficient, rather than overly robust, welfare program, which managed her trauma and abuse with a prescription pad.

Housing is a serious social issue in the Unites States. More than half of all Americans spend more than 30 percent of their income on housing, and many others spend over half of their income.[27] In 2019, a full-time worker earning minimum wage could not afford a two-bedroom apartment in any county in the United States, and only one in five households that qualified for federal housing assistance received it.[28] Without secure, safe, affordable housing, individuals cannot work, care for children, or survive. In such situations, medication is treated as a solution, but without other crucial support, medication could exacerbate and worsen underlying problems.

Betsy's story reflects institutional constraints faced by many doctors as well as their patients. For example, while talk therapy is reimbursed by insurance companies at incredibly low rates, prescribing drugs or performing a medical procedure is much more highly compensated.[29] Further, some doctors feel pressured to prescribe medication given their limited time with patients and inability to cure many of their patients who have chronic diseases. This is partially due to the fact that doctors who do not acquiesce to patients' demands run the risk of receiving low evaluations on hospital satisfaction surveys. Once they receive too many low scores, doctors are flagged in the system and risk losing their jobs.[30] Patients evaluate doctors more highly when they are provided with a treatment that shows a noticeable outcome, such as is the case with prescription drugs. In other words, both doctors and patients become ensnared in systems that promote the medicalization and pharmaceuticalization of ailments, causing everyone to suffer the consequences.

This chapter traced the stories of those who are trapped in a nexus of under- and over-treatment for physical, psychological, and emotional pain. Each of these stories began with pain. The medicalization—and pharmaceuticalization—of pain is offered as a means of treating symptoms without resolving the underlying causes. Suffering is thereby often exacerbated, as many of these interviewees developed a dependence on pharmacological substances—ones that contributed to arrest, incarceration, and devastation of their lives. Yet the likelihood of having one's experiences criminalized is not evenly distributed. Those who are already subject to greater state surveillance, on account of prior state custody in foster care, juvenile detention, rehabilitation centers, or prison, are also more likely to have their substance use criminalized. Those who come from more affluent backgrounds, who have higher education and greater access to quality, holistic health care, are also protected from state surveillance and punishment for compliance failure. It is precisely those who live in underfunded communities, who are under- or unemployed, and who are vulnerable to greater sources of stress and pain who are more likely to have their problems both medicalized and criminalized. They are also the individuals more likely be assigned labels that shape how their actions are perceived and treated. In the next chapter, I explore how this contributes to the prescription-to-prison pipeline.

3

PIPELINE

SORTING USE FROM ABUSE

Shaun was prescribed opioids to manage chronic knee and back pain after sustaining significant football injuries. He played football from a young age, all through high school, and even during his early years in college before his body finally gave out and he had to quit. It was devastating for him as football had been his life, but also because the pain was excruciating. Shaun, a forty-three-year-old Black man, describes how doctors often underprescribed medications to him because he was Black, and, he says, "not being dressed really nice or anything like that, [they assumed] that my sole intention was to come try to get medication to sell, and that wasn't the case." He describes how "the way that they treated me, it felt really bad. . . . They was really wrapped around trying to find reasons not to help me instead of figuring out what was wrong with me."

Shaun's story reflects a number of important intersectional issues related to race, gender, and class. Shaun sustained significant injuries as a result of playing football, a sport in which Black men are overrepresented. Football is a violent, full-contact sport in which players regularly sustain serious injuries, including concussions that can result in long-term brain damage. Injuries are so normalized in the sport that players learn early on not to complain, lest they have their playing time curtailed and risk their chances of being recruited to play on better teams. Shaun describes this experience exactly. Despite regular injuries, he rarely complained to anyone and went to a doctor only when the pain became unbearable with over-the-counter pain medication. He describes: "My knees were bad from football. I had Osgood-Schlatter," a condition that causes pain in the knee and upper shin when tendons pull against the top of the shinbone. Later, "[I] was put on prescription drugs again because my back had gotten bad, and I have a degenerative disease in my spinal cord." Despite these serious pain conditions, he felt as though the doctors regularly underprescribed medication to him while he was in pain. Friends suggested he try "some different pills like Amitriptyline, Xanax, and stuff like that," and so he did. He also tried marijuana. But then, at a routine doctor's appointment, Shaun's urine was tested without his knowledge. He was caught with marijuana in his system and stopped being prescribed medication entirely. His medical record became a criminal one.

Research finds that Black patients' descriptions of pain are taken less seriously by doctors, they are less likely to be prescribed opiates to manage pain than white patients, and those who receive opiates long term are more likely than white patients to be tested for illicit substance use. Of those who test positive, Black patients are also more likely than white patients to have their prescriptions discontinued.[1] Illicit substances that result in termination of medication include marijuana, for which Shaun screened positive. Although marijuana is now legally prescribed for patients with chronic pain and sold for recreational use in many states, at the time, its use, possession, or sale was still illegal.

After screening positive for marijuana, Shaun struggled with undermanaged chronic pain. He managed the pain through the intermittent prescriptions he received from doctors and smoking more marijuana. Shaun was arrested when "the police had kicked-in the house that I was at, and when they searched me, I had these pills in the cellophane, and of course, it's a felony to carry a controlled substance not in the prescribed bottle." He explains, "They were actually mine, I had a prescription for them. . . . I [even] brought the bottle to court, [but] it didn't help. I was in the wrong." Shaun was charged for the possession of a Schedule II substance (oxycodone) in addition to a Schedule I substance (marijuana).

Shaun grew up in a small town in central Missouri that was over 90 percent white and only 5 percent Black where "everybody knew everybody." Shaun and his three brothers were raised by his parents, who had been married for decades. Shaun's mother was always active in their local church, and, he says, "my brothers, all the men in my family side are military. My dad went to the military, my uncles went to the military. My grandpa went to the military. Everybody went to the military but me." Shaun's father had a stable union job, and, Shaun says, "we never did without. We always had everything we needed, utilities, water, clothes, food." That was why it was a shock that Shaun, and later his other brothers, ended up behind bars. He described how "it'd always be one of us in prison at a time, so it was like a big deal for my mom whenever all three of us were out for a holiday to make sure that we got together and have pictures and stuff, because it hurt her."

As a Black man in rural Missouri, Shaun was subject to particularly heightened police surveillance. He was more likely to be stopped and searched by police officers, which happened multiple times before his arrest. As one of the few Black students at his high school, Shaun stuck out in a lot of ways. A large, six-foot-five man, he described how he was expected to play football, a sport that consistently results in serious bodily harm. His experiences of being stopped and searched and of having doctors doubt his need or intention for using prescription drugs were also likely impacted by his race, class, and gender. As a Black man in the United States, Shaun is more likely to experience pain, to have his pain doubted, to be surveilled by doctors, to be searched by police officers, and to have his case prosecuted (and to be sentenced more harshly) than white counterparts, and less likely to receive quality health care and to receive legal counsel that could keep him out of prison.[2]

Shaun's story was not exceptional, as evidenced by the structural inequalities outlined above and as evidenced by the experiences of those interviewed for this book. Seventy percent (twenty-eight out of forty) of the women and 56 percent of the men (twenty-three out of forty) who were interviewed described how at least one of the prescription drugs that they used nonmedically had been initially prescribed to them by a doctor. All those who were interviewed were now sitting in prison, many of them on charges related to nonmedical prescription drug use as their "use" was eventually labeled as "abuse" by the police officers, judges, nurses, or doctors who wield the power to surveil and to classify.

Why did these individuals end up incarcerated when so many others use prescription drugs without intervention? This chapter focuses on the boundary work involved in delineating between legitimate and illegitimate substance use. It begins by highlighting the contradiction of a biologically defined concept of addiction as a "chronic, relapsing brain disease," whose diagnostic criteria remain at a behavioral level. Further, it highlights how these diagnostic criteria are informed by neoliberal, capitalist notions of well-being that conflate productivity with wellness and pleasure with illness. Moral judgment thus becomes codified in the medical gaze. Further, as a result of definitional ambiguity, classificatory systems such as the *Diagnostic and Statistical Manual of Mental Disorders* (DSM) afford undue power to those in control of diagnostic instruments or sentencing judgments. The result is that some groups—notably white, educated, upwardly mobile individuals—have the ability to navigate institutional spaces differently as a result of their social and cultural capital. In so doing, they evade the label of "addiction" or "abuse" and the associated consequences of being labeled a "criminal addict."

As sociologist Devah Pager argued in *Marked: Race, Crime, and Finding Work in an Era of Mass Incarceration*, the negative credential of a criminal record is directly linked with unemployment, homelessness, and recidivism itself. Unlike characteristics such as gender or race that are ascribed at birth, credentials—often conceived of in their positive form (e.g., college degrees or military service)—are often afforded greater weight in meritocratic societies such as the United States. The assumption is that someone has earned a credential, and that it therefore offers "a reasonable basis on which to determine status and access to opportunity" such as "jobs, housing, educational loans, welfare benefits, political participation, and other key social goods."[3]

This is similarly true for the negative credential, such as one's criminal or medical record, which has increasingly come to define one's trustworthiness and employability, as well as whether one deserves health care. Individuals with the negative credential of substance use are at even higher risk of incarceration if they have "two strikes" against them on account of a previous interaction with law enforcement or due to their race or class.[4] What this boils down to is that those who are already prone to greater state surveillance as a consequence of their race, class, gender, or involvement with state or child welfare programs are more likely to have their substance use constructed as abuse, a sign of addiction, or a "negative credential" warranting further state supervision and punishment.

"I Have an Addictive Personality": Biologizing
Behaviors through Diagnostic Labels

Addiction continues to be treated as a psychological disorder despite the fact that it has not been considered one for over twenty-five years. The last mention of addiction in the *DSM-III* was in 1986, when an international group of experts met to revise the section pertaining to substance-related disorders. It was removed on the grounds that the term *addiction* was "pejorative" and inconsistently used, thereby limiting its utility. As a consequence, *addiction* was replaced by the "more neutral term" *dependence*.[5] Despite this change, the term *addiction* continues to be used by health-care and legal practitioners as though it were a verifiable scientific reality. This results in inconsistent application, as the classification of one's use, in addition to one's treatment or punishment, is left to the individual discretion of doctors, pharmacists, or judges.

The most recent edition of the diagnostic manual, the *DSM-5*, combines categories of substance abuse and substance dependence to create a new diagnosis of a "substance use disorder" that is measured on a continuum from mild to severe.[6] While the diagnosis does not use the word *addiction*, its definition continues to be informed by the historical legacies of its religious and criminal predecessors, both of which were informed by white, middle-class notions of respectability and productivity. The *DSM-IV* was similar and offered the following definition for "substance abuse and substance dependence":

> A maladaptive pattern of substance use leading to clinically significant impairment or distress, as manifested by one (or more) of the following, occurring within a 12-month period:
> - Recurrent substance use resulting in a failure to fulfill major role obligations at work, school, or home (e.g., repeated absences or poor work performance related to substance use; substance-related absences, suspensions, or expulsions from school; neglect of children or household)
> - Recurrent substance use in situations in which it is physically hazardous (e.g., driving an automobile or operating machinery when impaired by substance use)
> - Recurrent substance-related legal problems (e.g., arrests for substance-related disorderly conduct)
> - Continued substance use despite having persistent or recurrent social or interpersonal problems caused or exacerbated by the effects of the substance (e.g., arguments with spouse about consequences of intoxication, physical fights)[7]

The fact that the definition hinges upon one's behavioral symptoms, including the "failure to fulfill major role obligations," "recurrent legal problems," or "persistent or recurrent social or interpersonal problems," reveals how defining addiction is intimately tied to existing economic, legal, and social structures. Such a definition implies that it is a psychological and biological problem if one is recurrently arrested by police officers or expelled by school administrators.

In the absence of genetic evidence of a disorder, behaviors (e.g., drug use, diagnosis of substance use disorder, arrest) are transformed into symptoms of underlying biology. Thus James, a fifty-one-year-old white man who dropped out of high school, believed that he was abusing prescription drugs because he had been arrested on such grounds, while his brother's nonmedical use was not abuse because he "was responsible, had a career." James also had steady employment before his arrest. With the aid of Xanax to manage his anxiety and OxyContin to provide energy, James made a good living as an arborist. James's substance use did not interfere negatively with his life until he was arrested. He had steady employment, housing, and a stabling living situation. Only after he was arrested did all that change. It was then that he picked up criminal charges as well as the diagnosis of "substance use disorder," which was the direct result of these criminal charges. Those without legal resources or who are subject to greater police surveillance run the risk of arrest and incarceration, in addition to a diagnosis of a medical disorder.

James's story and the DSM-5's criteria of dependence illustrate how medicalization compounds criminalization and vice versa. In so doing, it produces multiplicative effects of both institutions where some are doubly protected and others are doubly punished. For example, after describing his own so-called addiction, James contrasts his behavior with that of his older brother who "retired from [working for] the city after thirty years and never once ever had a problem in his legal life." James describes how much he respected and admired his older brother, who "was responsible, had a career," but then in the same breath describes him as a "chronic pill user." Because prescription drug use contributed to his brother's economic and social success in his career and with his family, it was difficult for James to see him as a "chronic, chronic, chronic opiate addict" as he saw himself.

James was introduced to opiates by his brother. However, because his brother was never arrested and charged for his nonmedical use nor sent to a rehabilitation program, James described his brother as an "upstanding guy," while he saw himself as both suffering from a disorder and having committed a crime. James draws upon the same circular logic used in official definitions of addiction: an individual is suffering from a substance use disorder or addiction if they have been arrested or sent to a rehabilitation program. The act of being arrested transforms one's use into abuse. Given what we know about uneven policing in the United States, it comes as no surprise that people of color who live in underresourced communities are more likely to be surveilled and arrested for their substance use. In the process, they are brought into a system that teaches them that recovery is impossible, that they suffer from a lack of willpower or are incapable of rational decision-making, or that addiction is a biological "brain disease" rather than socially produced. These myths are used to justify high rates of recidivism, the disenfranchisement of patients and prisoners, and punitive resocialization techniques of these institutions. Without the successful internalization of these myths, individuals and entities might reasonably question the efficacy of treatment programs and the very definition of substance abuse or addiction in the first place.

Such definitions conflate productivity with health and pleasure with disfunction and disease. The ability to uphold and legislate the binary between "productivity" and "pleasure" affords those in power, including doctors and judges, the power to designate certain behaviors or people as safe and others as dangerous. The Substance Abuse and Mental Health Services Administration (SAMHSA) and the National Institute on Drug Abuse (NIDA) define prescription drug misuse or abuse as "use without a prescription or solely for the feeling or experience caused by the drug." This is a similarly dangerous definition given that all substance use—prescription and nonprescription alike—is arguably for "the feeling or experience of the drug." Therefore, it remains up to the discretion of those diagnosing individuals, prescribing medication, or arresting, prosecuting, and sentencing individuals to decide the legitimacy of their substance use.

Legitimate substance use is bound up in notions of the gainfully employed, productive citizen. This is evidenced by the definitions offered by the DSM, SAMHSA, and NIDA, as well as those used by on-the-ground health-care practitioners, social workers, and employees at rehabilitation centers who teach patients how to interpret their behavior. All of those interviewed for this book attended rehabilitation programs prior to incarceration, and it was clear that many had internalized the labels and definitions employed by these programs, even in the absence of clear scientific operationalization. For example, most interviewees believed that using prescription drugs for pleasure or to "get high" was a sign of abuse or addiction. Jerome, a fifty-eight-year-old Black man, argues that he "abused" drugs because he used "for recreation, for fun, for feeling." Walter, a sixty-five-year-old Black man, similarly emphasized that abuse is when you "take them just for the hell of it. Just keep getting higher, and higher, and higher, and higher on the shit. Every day and every other day." For Jerome,

Walter, and many others, abuse is defined by the frequency of use as well as the intention—to have fun and get high rather than to work.

The medical definition of addiction locates the problem within an individual's brain rather than in the legal system that has outlawed a substance and that discriminates on the basis of race or class. This definition results in a more incisive and permanent diagnosis that can be undone only by a professional, which is troubling given that so many people become dependent upon substances as a result of a health-care professional.

The medical model of addiction caused interviewees to assume that there was something wrong with them rather than with the definition or the way such definitions are inconsistently applied. For example, Francis declares: "I crave bad. Why? I don't know. . . . [When I'm] told to go north, I go south. I've just always been that way." In regard to her convictions, she maintains, "I knew it was wrong, and I did it." Francis takes exclusive responsibility for her actions, attributing her drug use to her craving for "bad." She discounts other motivations for her drug use, such as the repeated sexual assaults and other abuse she experienced growing up. In doing so, she attributes her drug use and incarceration exclusively to her "addictive personality," which she perceives to be biological in nature.

Such framing causes us to misdirect treatment and solutions upon the individual or the drug, rather than upon the broader legal systems and environments. At first glance, conceiving of addiction as a "chronic, relapsing brain disease" rather than willful, deviant behavior may seem more humanistic. However, it actually extends the "corporeal gaze" focused on managing actions and bodies to a "neuro-molecular gaze" that seeks to reshape and control one's brain, which is more invasive and extreme.[8] The internalization of the addict diagnosis indicates the success of this shift, where individuals increasingly are convinced that they are imprisoned for neurological reasons rather than because of the system's overreliance upon pharmaceutical solutions. It also obscures the unevenness of these diagnoses and classifications. Those from higher classes, with higher education and greater cultural capital, may maneuver more easily between these labels and their associated consequences than those who are perpetually surveilled and policed.

"It's Not Illegal Drugs": Cultural Constructions of Prescription Medication

Off-label prescribing, where doctors prescribe a drug for a condition other than the one it has been approved for by the US Food and Drug Administration (FDA), is legal and common. Physicians defend this practice on the grounds that "it permits innovation in clinical practice" or "allows physicians to adopt new practices based on emerging evidence."[9] Yet, when individuals use prescriptions nonmedically (not entirely different from the practice of off-label prescribing), their use is constructed as abuse. This is because physicians and regulating bodies (e.g., the FDA) have the power to define what is use and what is abuse, while the patients are the subjects of this classification. It also reflects the stratified health-care system whereby some individuals have access to consistent quality care, in addition to association with medical professionals who can write them a script upon asking, whereas others lack access to both. This access results in not merely higher quality care but also a form of legitimacy that can justify and protect one's medicating habits.

Interviewees with greater cultural capital were more likely to perceive their prescription drug use as similar to off-label prescribing and had the means to justify that use, thereby protecting themselves from carceral intervention. Although the following case was somewhat unusual, it reflects an important example of how those with greater access and resources may be better insulated from the law.

When she was twelve, Irene tore her anterior cruciate ligament (ACL) and had to have surgery. The recovery took longer than expected, and she developed chronic pain from the resulting scar tissue. She was prescribed pain medication by her surgeon and took the pills intermittently to manage the pain. She ended up having to have another reconstructive surgery years later, for which she was again prescribed opiates. Following that, Irene had two more knee surgeries and eight other surgeries for a variety of ailments, including a host of gallbladder issues and an abscessed brown recluse spider bite. Across these surgeries, Irene, a twenty-nine-year-old white woman, had been prescribed oxycodone, OxyContin, Darvocet, Tylenol with codeine, Vicodin, Lortab, Lorcet, and Percocet.

Irene's mother was a nurse. Whenever Irene had a surgery and her prescription ran out, her mother would often "know the doctor, so she would tell the doctor and they would prescribe [more] narcotics." Her mother didn't want Irene to be in pain, and she used her resources to help. This provided Irene access to prescription drugs whenever she needed. When I asked Irene if her mother knew that she often took more pills than she was prescribed, Irene says, "Yeah, my mom did. She always knew. . . . She looks at it differently because, like I said, she's a nurse, so in her mind it's not illegal drugs." From her mother's perspective, prescription drugs are medicine, even if they're not used exactly as prescribed by a doctor. Irene's mother is not unique in this respect. People who are prescribed opiates by their doctors and become unable to stop are diagnosed as "drug dependent" or "tolerant" rather than "addicted." Further, patients who use opiates nonmedically tend to be viewed with greater empathy by doctors than those who use illicit substances.[10] As a member of the medical field herself, Irene's mother saw the distinction between medical and nonmedical use of a medication as arbitrary. The important distinction was between licit and illicit substances, despite their many chemical similarities.

Although Irene was not a nurse herself, growing up middle class and with regular access to doctors and interactions with her mother's colleagues, she learned how to talk to doctors in convincing ways. She explains, "When you can talk the doctor talk, which I was, like I said, raised in a medical family, then they like that and they're like, 'Oh OK, well obviously you know what's wrong with you,' and they just write a prescription." This fluency allows people like Irene to be treated as part of this privileged class and obtain access to the pharmacological capital associated with it. This harks back to nineteenth-century physicians who were disproportionately likely to be addicted to opiates, given that those with greatest access to medical care are often the ones at greatest risk for dependence.[11]

The risks of using prescription drugs nonmedically are less severe for the white, middle and upper classes given that they are less frequently policed, have greater ability to afford legal representation, and thus are less likely to face incarceration. This may account for why interviewees perceived that nonmedical prescription drug use is more common among "the higher classes" (Shaun), "more professional people" (Diana), or "cops, doctors, lawyers. A lot of people that are higher up in your community that you wouldn't think would be doing them or selling them and people that you would look at like 'Oh, they don't use drugs'" (Yasmin). Individuals who live in more affluent communities are often insulated from policing and punishment and have greater access to doctors and health care.

Jaclyn, a thirty-year-old white woman, describes how "the rich folks" can more easily "get a prescription from the doctor" or even "buy the pills . . . [and] say that they're not getting high." She describes how they "don't get in trouble because [they can say] it's the prescription I was prescribed. . . . They don't lose their job, they don't get in trouble." Jaclyn adeptly identifies the associated privilege of one's social class (in addition to race) that protects them from the types of consequences faced by many of those interviewed for this study.

The perception that prescription drug use is more common among the affluent reflects the successful boundary work accomplished by politicians, lawyers, doctors, pharmacists, and the criminal justice system to establish prescription drugs as safe, legal medications used with the intention to cure legitimate ailments and other drugs as dangerous, illicit substances used with the intention to get high. Given disparities in access to health care, nonmedical prescription drug use or "pill popping" reflects a type of cultural capital, and association with medical professionals—even as merely a patient seeing a doctor—becomes a form of social capital. In combination, medical and nonmedical prescription drug use has come to be associated with white, middle and upper classes even as their use has become more widespread.[12]

This conceptual distinction impacts both perception and behavior. For example, Diana, a thirty-three-year-old white woman who attended college, describes how "most of my family, they take a pill for something. A pill for that and a pill for that, you know? Because it's legal." She goes on to clarify that "if it's legal, it's all right, you know, the state says it is. America says it is. Illegal means that the law says—My mom and dad were law-abiding citizens. My mom wouldn't—If it said forty-five miles per hour, she wouldn't do forty-six or forty-seven. But yet, she'd do all the dope she wanted to because it was legal." In college, Diana witnessed many upwardly mobile students using prescription drugs who, like her parents, did not believe it was dangerous.

Prescription drug use was often perceived to be safer and less harmful because it often began in a doctor's office. However, whose use constitutes medical use and whose is abuse is often tied to social location. While some are insulated from the law as a result of their race, class, or gender, others face greater scrutiny. Specifically, those who had already been classified once as an "addict," "foster youth," or "juvenile delinquent" were more likely to be further policed and punished. In contrast, those with the institutional capital of a medical degree were more likely to be trusted and insulated from legal action.

"An Addict Don't Make Sense Anyways": Discounting Embodied Knowledge

When asked why she would combine prescription drugs with one another, Georgia, a twenty-seven-year-old white woman, jokes, "'Cause it says not to on the bottle?" and laughs. She follows up by explaining that if "someone doesn't have a drug problem, then they would actually [follow] that stuff." In response to the same question, Janice, a thirty-nine-year-old white woman, replies, "I don't know why they'd mix them, maybe meth because you're so high-strung and Xanax just makes you immortal. [But] no, it don't make sense, no. An addict don't make sense anyways. Nothing we do makes sense." Despite Georgia and Janice's self-deprecation, the rationale they each offered to explain why someone would combine substances was both reasonable *and* ideologically aligned with medical (as well as neoliberal) discourse—to mitigate effects and to increase productivity. And yet they discounted their own expertise as coming from "addicts" with "a drug problem," as they have been trained to do.

Almost half of the people interviewed referred to themselves as an "addict" or "junkie" at some point during the interview—labels or "negative credentials" that carry powerful consequences in medical and legal contexts.[13] Similar to the way that employers "appear less concerned about specific information conveyed by a criminal conviction and its bearing on a particular job, but rather view this credential as an indicator of general employability or trustworthiness," one's medical or legal substance use record similarly "comes to stand for a broader internal disposition."[14] The frequency with which interviewees spontaneously used this language to describe themselves reflects how fundamental this discourse is to justifying and legitimizing our interviewees' punishment. It also highlights how the power to control lies in the ability to distinguish use from abuse or medical from nonmedical use of prescription drugs.

Individuals with a documented history of substance use are treated differently in a health-care setting than those without; they may be subject to greater surveillance or have their access to medications curtailed.[15] Those identified and labeled as a "drug seeker" by the health-care system are the targets of social and institutional discrimination.[16] This diagnostic label not only creates a barrier to comprehensive medical care but also increases the likelihood that the individual will be criminally charged for substance use. Even if the individual is not convicted of criminal charges, such involvement with the criminal legal system can significantly affect their life, with consequences such as losing custody of their children or being barred from certain employment or housing opportunities.

Stacey, a thirty-two-year-old white woman, describes how doctors treated her differently because of her history of substance use. She describes how doctors "don't ask me no questions" and rarely prescribe her medications. She attributes her poor treatment to the fact that she was "airlifted to a hospital because I was in a meth lab house fire." As a result, doctors "just assume I'm a drug addict—which, I mean, I *am* a drug addict"—and therefore don't listen to her, do not believe her symptoms, and will undermedicate her when she is in pain. Stacey believes that her care is inadequate as a result of how she is perceived by doctors; however, by claiming "I *am* a drug addict," she expresses her own internalization of the label and diagnosis as well.

The label of "addict" may lower levels of trust between patient and health-care provider, which could ironically increase the likelihood of nonmedical prescription drug use.[17] For example, Raphael, a forty-two-year-old white man, describes how he is treated differently by doctors as a result of having a medical and criminal record of using illicit substances. He describes how he is "from a small town, [and] the doctor I had is one of the only ones around. He knew my history as far as being a drug addict and stuff. So he's not going to give me Xanaxes or Valiums, even if I might need them, he's not even going to consider that. He's going to think, 'Oh he's trying to get drugs!' You know?" Raphael suffers from anxiety, which he says keeps him from being able to sleep or focus when he's awake. However, the doctor in his town was reticent to prescribe him anything due to his criminal history. As a result, he's been forced to find alternative ways to get medication or treatment—ways that added more pages to his criminal record.

This catch-22, where individuals who need medications are denied them as a result of former run-ins with law enforcement over the very medications they need, was common among our interviewees. For example, Oscar, a thirty-seven-year-old white man, was diagnosed with attention deficit hyperactivity disorder (ADHD) as a teenager and used to medicate regularly under a doctor's supervision. However, per a recommendation from a friend, he started mixing his Ritalin medication with methamphetamines to amplify its effects. Unbeknownst to him, his urine was tested at a routine doctor's visit and he came up positive for meth. After that, his prescription for Ritalin was terminated. He explains how once "you've got a record of abusing drugs, they usually don't prescribe you anything. I know 'cause I got ADHD and I can't get no ADHD meds." Oscar's ADHD inhibits his ability to focus and to do the things he both needs and wants to do. The criteria for addiction include the "failure to fulfill major role obligations at work, school, or home," but Ritalin was what enabled Oscar to work and take care of his family. Yet, his diagnosis as an "addict" trumps that of his ADHD, thus dictating his medical treatment.

"I Have to Trust Them . . . Because I'm Not a Doctor":
Privileging Professionals

Interviewees had complex relationships with both doctors and the field of medicine. When asked if they trusted doctors, over a third of interviewees said they did not. An additional third struggled to respond to the question, offering explanations such as "I don't trust doctors, but I trust the profession." Respondents struggled to form opinions that challenged the prevailing cultural narrative that people with greater education are necessarily more qualified and trustworthy. Even when doctors prescribed medicine and treatment that were ineffective or harmful, some interviewees continued to trust the doctor's authority over their own. You can hear this tension expressed by Evan, a forty-one-year-old white man, when he discussed whether he trusts doctors: "I think for the most part, most of them are very smart—I think most of them are there for—I mean that's what they—I don't know, yeah, I trust them, just because I haven't had any bad experiences, I guess. I mean, I think if you go to school, go to college and all that stuff, and you make it that far in life, I think evidently you're dedicated to something. I mean—." Harry, a forty-two-year-old white man, offers a similar explanation for trusting doctors: "If they went through that much school and they're smart enough to even do that, they gotta know something." These responses reflect a culture that constructs doctors as eternally ethical, well-intentioned, and omniscient rather than fallible humans.

James, a fifty-one-year-old white man, articulates the struggle eloquently: "I have to trust them, that's the only thing, because I'm not a doctor. I'm not professional in the field of medicine or the anatomy of the body, so I have to pretty much . . . I have to accept it because that's all I got, it's nothing else there. But a doctor to me, he's just a glorified drug pusher as far as I'm concerned." Despite negative personal experiences with doctors and the characterization of doctors as "glorified drug pushers," James continues to respect the profession of medicine, in part because of the associated credentials. He explains, "That's all I got," indicating that he does not have the medical education to discern his problem or an appropriate treatment, so he is forced to rely on those who have the education and status in society of "doctor." And yet, when individuals do attempt to identify and solve problems on their own, they run the risk of criminalization—a fact that forcibly tells people they require medical and legal oversight.

Others were openly distrustful of a medical system that seemed more interested in categorically classifying and medicating them according to a disorder than in trying to understand the complexities of their social conditions. Such was the case for Alejandro, a fifty-three-year-old white and Native American man, who believed that he had been prescribed psychotropics as a means of subduing and controlling his behavior. He described how the pills he'd been prescribed made him "sleep too much, and feel groggy" but that his care team would say, "'Oh, he's better now, he's asleep.' Get the hell outta here." He went on: "I really just feel like they're doing experiments on you, you know what I mean?"

Access to health care, including type and duration, is impacted by one's social location. In the United States, one must pay for one's health care, and being able to do so reflects significant privilege that can significantly impact one's life outcomes. While programs like Medicaid and Medicare make health care more accessible to those who have historically been priced out of coverage, poorly funded health care often fails to provide comprehensive preventive physical and mental health care programs, which results in more liberal prescription of psychotropics rather than alternative treatment or support.

This was the experience of Betsy, the thirty-three-year-old white woman introduced in chapter 2. When she was seventeen, Betsy went to see a psychiatrist and said she was having anxiety and depression. "I was on Medicaid. Bam, just like that, Xanax here you go, just wrote me a prescription. He didn't even listen to what I said, didn't care." Betsy attributes her subsequent substance use to that experience and to inferior health care accessed through Medicaid. She explains, "I'm sure that there [are] good doctors out there. I wouldn't know nothing about that because I've always been on Medicaid and to be completely honest, I've never been to a good doctor or a good psychiatrist for that matter." She attributes her lack of quality care to the fact that "this world is corrupt and I think government is corrupt and I think Medicaid is a joke. They don't help. They don't want to help, they just want to make money. That's just the truth, that's just the way it is. You've got money, you've got a good job, you have insurance, you're going to see a good doctor." Without money or a job with good benefits, you are less likely to receive comprehensive care.

Similarly, Paul, a fifty-five-year-old man of Black, Indigenous, and European heritage, described how doctors never listened to him; instead, they were eager to ascribe a label and prescribe an associated medication. He describes how he had "been prescribed psychotropic drugs" since his early thirties "for my manic depression, my schizoid disorders, what they call it." He explains how frustrating it is when he is "telling the truth about things that's really happened" to him but that doctors treat him as though he is "delusional or paranoid schizophrenic" as a way to discount his reality. At other times, he describes how when he was "kind of sad, now [he is] manic depressant, and yet you didn't really do no kind of in-depth interview or see what's going on." From Paul's perspective, the doctors are "automatically just giving me a title and give me some pills and say, 'Here, go on.' They just listen to a little bit of it and, you know, boom. 'This is what's wrong with you.'" Without their getting to know his story individually, he felt reduced to a diagnostic label or criminal charge.

It was clear from these interviews that many felt neglected by doctors and the field of medicine more broadly. As a result, they felt better off determining their own course of treatment through self-medication rather than seeking a specialist who "ain't got no time for you." That was how Kevin, a forty-seven-year-old white man who dropped out of high school and has been arrested over one hundred times, described his experiences. He was institutionalized when he was "eleven or twelve," but, he says, "both times I escaped and ran away" because "they would put me in a rubber room and shoot [medication] in my butt." Kevin believed that he needed medication as a child, but it felt punitive and violent in its administration. He also believes that even if he had been diagnosed earlier, that may not have deterred him from getting into trouble, given that he believes that some of the medications he was prescribed turned him into "a drug addict." He argues that "the whole world's [on] drugs out there now, 'You need this, here take these, take these, take these.' A little too much I think." And yet Kevin often didn't use the medication he was prescribed because "mom and dad I don't think could afford them when we were kids." As a result, he used marijuana to help manage withdrawal symptoms from his medication. His marijuana was grounds for arrest and incarceration, thus solidifying both "addict" and "criminal" identities.

Health-care and legal practitioners regulate access to prescription drugs via a moral economy. While medicine and the criminal legal system are treated as distinct institutions, they work in tandem to police pleasure, determining whose needs are legitimate and whose are illegitimate. As sociologist Liz Chiarello argues, health-care practitioners must make "medical, legal, and moral assessments" in their diagnoses and treatment. These "tactics constitute mechanisms of policing pleasure by controlling those resources that facilitate pleasure while assessing the moral worthiness of specific patients."[18]

The regulation of pleasure is directly tied to cultural definitions of productivity and moral worthiness. Arguably, all pain and medical relief is an inherently pleasure-seeking aspiration; however, health-care practitioners remain the arbiters of the proper use of substances, which is tied to definitions of health and normalcy that are marked by heightened productivity, discipline, and self-regulation.[19]

In the next chapter, I complete the prescription-to-prison-pipeline circuit by highlighting how labels of addiction and abuse have been bound up in diagnostic labels of mental illness and legal identifications of criminality. I argue that such classificatory systems entrap individuals in a repetitive feedback loop where individuals are medicalized and criminalized by drug courts, rehabilitation programs, prisons, probation, and parole ad infinitum. Individuals are expected to relapse and recidivate—and they often do.

4

PRISON

FROM MEDICALIZATION TO CRIMINALIZATION

The very first woman I interviewed for this project was a fifty-four-year-old Black woman named Andrea. Andrea was expelled from grade school when she was thirteen years old. At that point, she had already been suspended from school numerous times. When she was eighteen, she was diagnosed by a doctor as suffering from paranoid schizophrenia, and she was prescribed an assortment of prescription drugs, including Darvocet, Clonazepam, Vicodin, Percocet, and OxyContin. On the recruitment survey about nonmedical prescription drug use, Andrea indicated that she had used each of these prescription drugs nonmedically. She was selected for an interview because, based on her survey responses, she seemed to have considerable experiences to share.

However, early on in the interview, Andrea seemed confused. When I asked basic questions about her substance use or life experiences, she couldn't seem to understand what I was asking. She also could not find the words to respond when she did understand the questions. It was not clear if this was the result of cognitive issues or the effects of sedative medication. Either way, it did not seem right to continue.

Andrea has been locked up for most of her life—arrested fourteen times over the course of her life—and was most recently incarcerated on charges of drug possession and theft.[1] When I asked her why she was incarcerated, she seemed confused. Andrea couldn't explain the circumstances that led to her arrest. I decided to stop the interview early. Someone can consent to participating in a study only if they fully understand the study, including its potential risks and harms. I was losing confidence that the consent Andrea provided was truly informed, and it felt inappropriate to be talking to her about her experience if she could not comprehend what was going on. I was unsettled. This was the first interview of the project; I wondered whether I would be able to conduct any interviews as I would not continue with an interview that went similarly to Andrea's. However, it was even more troubling that Andrea was locked up in a prison cell rather than living in a home or facility that could provide her with adequate mental health support and not sedate her with medication.

Andrea's story is much too common. Between 1955 and 2016, the number of hospital beds in state psychiatric institutions dropped 97 percent.[2] Meanwhile, the total number of incarcerated people (including those with serious mental illnesses) has more than tripled. While the United States incarcerated 209 people per 100,000 in 1978, by 2018, that number had jumped to 706 per 100,000; roughly 2.3 million people were behind bars.[3] In fact, one study of data from 2004 to 2005 found that there were triple the number of individuals with serious mental health issues in jails and prisons than in hospitals; in another study conducted in 2012, ten times as many.[4]

The shuttering of mental hospitals has left a gap in health services, particularly for those like Andrea who have experienced emotional and psychological trauma from a young age and who lack the appropriate support. Prescription drugs have become the centerpiece of mental health care, particularly for the incarcerated and others in institutionalized settings such as foster care or juvenile detention.[5] Prescription drugs, notably psychotropics, are often the *only* mental health treatment available to incarcerated people.[6] Further, as nonpharmaceutical mental health services (e.g., psychotherapy) are only minimally reimbursed by health insurance, psychotropics are increasingly the only accessible option. Psychotropic treatment has become coercive in situations where psychiatric treatment is part of the incarceration process or a mandated condition of probation or parole. This can feed into a punishing feedback loop whereby the medications prescribed as a condition of parole later serve as a violation of that parole when individuals use them nonmedically. This is particularly common among those who are subject to greater policing and punishment, such as those in poor, nonwhite neighborhoods or under government supervision (e.g., foster care or juvenile detention).

In his book *Silent Cells: The Secret Drugging of Captive America*, sociologist Anthony Hatch traces how psychotropics are an essential technology in subduing and controlling institutionalized populations, such as those in foster care, nursing homes, the military, and, most significantly, prisons.[7] He argues that the control and pacification of the millions of incarcerated people are possible *because* of the regular administration of psychotropics. This practice may also sow seeds of distrust in medicine. This is significant given that distrust is a major contributing factor to the nonmedical use of prescription drugs and thereby may ultimately contribute to the prescription-to-prison pipeline. Thus the circuit completes itself: the overprescription of certain populations results in dependence, but also distrust. Backed into a corner, they must obey the doctor or run the risk of criminalization and reinstitutionalization.

In this chapter, I explore the effects of deinstitutionalization and transinstitutionalization on individuals like Andrea who need support rather than punishment. All our interviewees were mandated to attend a rehabilitation program prior to their incarceration. Drawing upon other studies of therapeutic jurisprudence and court-mandated rehabilitation programs, I highlight how pernicious discourses of the criminal addict have been internalized by interviewees in ways that may do significant harm to their self-concept and mental health. As a result, such programs may in fact perpetuate greater substance use or harmful behavior as interviewees have already been labeled and cast aside by social institutions. Further, as reintegration into society becomes a challenge for those who have become disenfranchised, medication is often a primary coping mechanism, as well as a risk factor for recidivism.

"I'm Just an Addict": Labeled into the System

Over fifty percent of incarcerated people in the United States have been diagnosed with a mental health disorder.[8] In our interviews, a quarter of the men (nine out of forty) and fifty percent of the women (twenty out of forty) had been diagnosed with a psychiatric disorder, and many of them had been prescribed psychotropics.[9] The fact that those in need of medical attention are housed in a prison rather than receiving mental health support and treatment is likely attributable to the twin pillars of deinstitutionalization of mental health care and transinstitutionalization between mental health facilities and prisons.

Deinstitutionalization is the term used to describe the shift of mental health care away from mental health institutions, most readily identified by the shrinking number of mental health care facilities. Most notably, by the year 2000, the number of state hospital beds for those with mental health issues had dropped from its peak in 1955 of 339 per 100,000 people to just 22 per 100,000 people on any given day.[10] Alongside this trend, the United States has witnessed increased transinstitutionalization: the transfer of the individuals from mental health facilities to other institutions, such as prisons, foster care, and nursing homes.[11] This is evidenced by the fact that between 1978 and 2000, the number of incarcerated people with mental illness increased from 209 to 708 per 100,000 people.[12] Transinstitutionalization is the direct consequence of deinstitutionalization: as mental hospitals are shut down, many suffering from mental trauma end up in jails and prisons, foster care, or nursing homes, or on the streets, where they learn to cope with a combination of prescription and illicit substances.

Deinstitutionalization was the result of both fiscal conservativism of the 1980s, which resulted in drastic cuts to mental and physical health-care programs, and successful civil rights efforts to humanize and destigmatize mental health care. While mental hospitals provided wraparound care via therapy, medication, work, vocational training, and community, they also were environments for considerable abuse and disenfranchisement, especially given that many people—those deemed mentally unfit—were confined without consent. Disability rights activists successfully fought for the rights of those who were confined and treated against their will. Without an alternative, or sufficient state or federal funding, many of those with serious mental illness have ended up without treatment or the ability to afford housing, food, or other basic necessities given that Supplemental Security Income provided by the Aid to Disabled Program provides an income that is well below the poverty line.[13]

Equally as troubling, a number of studies have demonstrated how those struggling with mental health often become entrenched in the criminal justice system: they stay incarcerated longer given that they are less likely to be released under community supervision and are almost twice as likely to "have their probation or parole revoked and return to jail or prison than others charged with similar offenses."[14] These trends reflect multiple mechanisms underlying the prescription-to-prison pipeline, whereby (1) medical diagnoses are increasingly blurred with criminal ones (e.g., addiction, substance use disorder), (2) without adequate social, financial, or political support, individuals end up in prisons rather than in supportive communities, and (3) individuals have social and structural problems addressed through medication, often in institutionalized settings such as prisons, and are later penalized for that very drug use that was initiated by physicians or more broadly supported by medical and neoliberal discourse.

One of the primary diagnoses that contributes to transinstitutionalization might be that of addiction. As the social pariah, the "criminal addict" *requires* medical treatment, carceral punishment, and public scrutiny. Their drug use is *at risk* of harming others, even if it has not already. In other words, criminal addicts are *risky subjects* or *at risk* of becoming troublesome. And this risk warrants and justifies perpetual surveillance, such as is commonplace in rehabilitation and treatment centers, juvenile detention facilities, and prisons.

"I've Been Locked Up Off and On My Entire Life": Institutional Entrapment

Rachel, a twenty-seven-year-old white woman, has spent the majority of her life in institutionalized care: shuffled from a psychiatric hospital to a juvenile detention center to foster care and finally to prison, where I met her. While in labor with Rachel, her mother suffered a stroke, leaving her body paralyzed. As a result, her father had to care for both his newborn daughter and his wife. This took an emotional toll on both parents as well as Rachel. When Rachel was nine years old, her "dad committed suicide in front of" her, an event that Rachel still has difficulty processing. When she was eleven, she was "hospitalized for depression and stuff." While hospitalized, Rachel was prescribed a number of psychotropic medications to manage her mental health. She continued to use them after being released to her mother's care. However, between "eleven and twelve I got locked up for stealing bikes and stuff. I started going to juvenile and foster homes and in and out of my mom's life." During this time, Rachel's mother started using her own pain medication in greater quantities and combined it with other illicit substances such as cocaine and methamphetamines. She pushed Rachel to take the pills with her so she wouldn't be using on her own. Rachel was fourteen. At fifteen, Rachel got pregnant and delivered via a cesarean section, which resulted in prescriptions for "Percocets and Hydros. Something else for muscle relaxing . . . I get prescribed all those, and then I end up having a hemorrhoidal surgery. I got double the Percocets and Hydros." Rachel didn't like how the medications made her feel, but she did know that she could sell them for good money. As a single working mother, that helped her cover some of the bills. But Rachel was arrested and charged for selling them. As she describes, "I've been locked up off and on my whole life."

Rachel's story illustrates the reverberating impacts of trauma, but also how state intervention can exacerbate these effects. Her experiences—the trauma of her mother's paralysis and substance use, her father's suicide, the poverty she experienced growing up—were medicalized early on. But she never felt as though the doctors were there to help. Rachel says "psychiatrists and stuff, I really think are a bunch of quacks" who give you drugs and "send you on your way." Rachel's interaction with the health-care system was cold and impersonal and predominantly took the form of prescriptions, many of which resulted in future incarceration.

Childhood trauma, psychiatric treatment, and juvenile detention centers are often the beginning of a long cycle through the state criminal justice system, or what sociologist Beth Richie calls a "prison nation"[15] apparatus, which includes probation, parole, home supervision, welfare, child protective services, or other forms of frequent state intervention and subsequent policing. Once an individual becomes part of the prison nation apparatus, it can be difficult to become disentangled from it. This was true for a number of our interviewees.

Of the nine interviewees we spoke to who grew up in foster care, five had also been in juvenile detention centers and one in a psychiatric inpatient clinic. For example, Diana, a thirty-three-year-old white woman, describes how she started using drugs at a young age and as a result ended up in a juvenile detention center. "As a juvenile, I was placed in group homes because of my behavior. Basically, I got put on probation and I kept running away from home, so my parents called the cops and then I'd get put in a group home. I kept running from those." Patrick, a fifty-seven-year-old Native American man, similarly describes how he has gone "through foster homes, boys' prison, detention, all through my whole life."

Children who grow up in the foster care system experience considerable hardships compared to those who do not. As many as one in three will experience a period of homelessness by age twenty-six.[16] Education and employment rates are well below those of other low-income individuals, as well as the general population, and between 20 and 60 percent will be involved in the carceral system within two years of leaving the foster system.[17]

Patrick was one of those children who grew up in the foster care system and whose life trajectory maps onto these statistics. He describes how he "was in a car wreck with my mom when I was four months old and she died. I had severe head injuries. I almost didn't make it through." Patrick survived the accident, but his mother's death was difficult on his father. His father worked on the railroad and was often gone. He remarried soon after his wife's death and left Patrick with his new wife, who was abusive. In addition to suffering physical abuse from his stepmother, Patrick describes how his father "knocked my teeth out and he did things to me. Then one of his friends molested me." After many years of abuse, Patrick was transferred to foster care, later to a boys' home, and eventually to a juvenile detention center after being arrested and charged for possession of illicit substances.

Patrick describes the experience of being molested, raped, and shuffled between institutions as both devastating and isolating. He coped with low self-esteem and mental trauma by using opioids to manage pain and help him sleep. He would take them in the middle of the night to get just a few hours of sleep before work. But then he was too groggy the next day, so he "got addicted to methamphetamine. That took over." He was caught in possession of meth and sent to prison. "Then I got raped in prison, when I first went to prison. That flipped my mind around to where it just made me go into a dark, dark area of my life. It stayed that way for years until probably a few years ago."

Patrick suffered his entire life, first at the hands of his father and later at the hands of the state that failed to care for and protect him. His story is all too common, whereby children in foster care or juvenile detention rarely get the "second chance" they are promised. Instead, they are transported between homes, facilities, and detention centers where they rarely receive the support they need. Instead of receiving treatment for childhood traumas, he was confined to a series of punitive institutions where his problems were medicalized, often being constructed as biological rather than the product of social inequities. The failure of social services in facilitating community reintegration often results in long-term institutionalization (e.g., foster care, juvenile detention, prison).[18]

This story of bouncing between foster homes is sadly a common one in the United States. More than half a million children in the United States are serviced by the foster care system in any given year.[19] Of those children, less than 5 percent returned to the place they called home prior to foster care. Approximately one-third of them (32 percent) are placed in the home of a family member, and a little under half are adopted by a nonrelative (45 percent). However, 17 percent of foster children are never placed in a permanent family home, instead living in an institutional setting or being shuffled between foster homes. Children who age out of foster care without a permanent home or family have much higher incidences of poverty, homelessness, and incarceration. As a result of this instability, a significant proportion of children in the foster care system will end up involved with the criminal justice system within a few years of aging out.[20]

This was the case with Quentin, a fifty-eight-year-old white man, who also grew up in foster care. He describes how "my dad died before I met him" and "my mom was a gypsy. She gave me away when I was eight years old. . . . My mom was pregnant with me and there was three of us and she kept me until I was eight. She gave my oldest brother away when he was in diapers." After that, he had "been in foster homes, and foster homes, and foster homes, you know?" He describes how "some of them were bad, some of them were good. Some of them were just for the check. Some of them weren't. Most all of them were for the check." Much of his medical care felt similar to this experience—where he was less often treated as a human and more often as a financial liability. He recalls:

> I lived a rough life, you know? I've been shot, stabbed, all that's good for pain pills. Go to the doctor, hospital and—I was in a hunting accident, buddy of mine shot me in the side of the leg, and they doped me up in the hospital. Appendix, doped me up in the hospital. Gave me lots of pills when I got out. They cracked a rib because my appendix was up here instead of down here. When they pried it open, they made a mistake and scratched my lung and cracked a rib. Therefore triple more pain and I had to stay in the hospital longer instead of having the appendix out, out the next day three or four days. They said, "Oh, don't sue us. Here's a piece of paper and we will give you all the pain medicine you want." They did, ninety Percocet right out the door and paid for.

Quentin became dependent upon opioids. He used them for years until his prescription ran out. At that point he started using heroin, which was cheaper and more accessible to him. He is currently serving time on charges related to his heroin use. Quentin had good reason to distrust doctors, yet he was the one who was treated as untrustworthy by medical and legal systems, in large part because of his substance use and his associated diagnostic and criminal labels that have increasingly blurred together conceptually and practically.

*"We're Always Going to Be Junkies": Genetic
and Criminal Essentialism*

Increasingly, addiction is conceived of as a neurological disease rather than a moral failing. However, the medicalization of addiction has arguably afforded moralizing judgment even *more* power. On the surface, instruments and technologies that can identify and visualize disorders appear to destigmatize and legitimize these experiences, as well as to construct those labels as objective "facts."[21] Yet as a result these diagnoses take on greater permanence and therefore greater stigmatization. They also erase the interpretive human element involved. For example, people are increasingly likely to attribute depression or schizophrenia to neurobiology rather than to inaccessible economic and social structures or individual proclivities.[22] However, attributing a disorder to one's genes has the effect of establishing those suffering to "seem more fundamentally different than others" and reduce the possibility for change.[23]

This conceptual move negates the possibility for recovery as the person *becomes* the diagnosis rather than someone living with one. Although some attribution theorists believed that reducing one's causal responsibility for an illness might reduce its stigma, *genetic essentialism* actually ties the person ever more closely to the illness. The consequences for individuals diagnosed as suffering from addiction or dependence may be even more extreme, as they experience simultaneous *genetic* and *criminal essentialism* and are therefore incapable of escaping their biology or recurrent treatment (if they're lucky) and incarceration (if they aren't).

Many of the individuals interviewed believed that addiction was their biological destiny and that it was untethered from substances specifically. For example, both Lauren and Gina traced their addiction to their families, arguing that addiction had been passed down to them biologically. Lauren, a thirty-year-old white woman, describes how "my family's pretty screwed up. There's a lot of addicts." Similarly, Gina, a forty-four-year-old Black woman, insists that it's in her blood; she relates, "My maternal grandmother was an alcoholic, still is today. My mom has a gambling addiction." Both of their responses imply that addiction is a biological trait, something that could be passed down from a grandmother or mother. To Gina, drinking, gambling, and drug use are all related and tied to the broader trait of addiction. By grouping these actions together, a child of a gambler should be wary of alcohol, drugs, sex, or anything else deemed addictive by our society given an "at risk" biological predisposition.

For those who identified as an addict or junkie, most described it as a permanent diagnosis: "We're always going to be junkies." For example, Steve laments that "a junkie is a junkie." While he describes wanting to change, Steve argues that when you're a junkie, you are "going to keep using until you're tired of using. You might get on and try to get in a program and do what you want to do, until you get out there on the streets and then everything's there." There is a sense of hopelessness to their accounts as they insist that addiction is part of their biology and therefore an inescapable fate.

Patrick describes himself as "addicted" to "criminal activity," describing how "you would feel so bold just to steal anything at any time." He describes how breaking the law "invoked that superman mentality. That was part of my addiction with that. I just could hide and cover up and be somebody I wasn't." In explaining why he used drugs, Patrick refers to his father, who "could drink a gallon of whiskey and sit down and just talk to you like it was normal. My thing would be like, that much in drugs. I was an addict, and I was a severe one." Instead of focusing on his traumatic childhood, when he was molested and shuffled between abusive families in foster care, or the fact he was raped in prison, Patrick attributes his incarceration to his biology, as indicated by his father's alcoholism.

Patrick is also convinced that he is a repeat offender because he is addicted to prison. He has been arrested "seven hundred or so" times for charges "related to drugs." From his perspective, "doing time in prison becomes addicting. I'll just go back to prison, no big deal. I know how to do that real good." However, in the same breath that he claims to be addicted to prison, he grieves his "desire to get out there and work with young kids. I wanna go to college and I wanna learn social studies and I wanna take Bible school. My thing is, I wanna work with young men, young guys. Those are the future of our country." Somehow, his hopes and intentions are minimized by a deterministic biological logic in which he will always be an addict and incarcerated man. His narrative discounts the many barriers faced by the incarcerated when they are released from prison, such as being barred from affordable housing, educational loans, or other social services such as food and medical assistance. Instead of focusing on the structural barriers and environmental traumas that have shaped his psyche and actions, he looks inward to his biological or moral constitution as the explaining variables of his life.

Paralleling anthropologist Angela Garcia's findings in *The Pastoral Clinic*, interviewees discussed their drug use with such resignation, reiterating the dominant explanatory model used by scientists and caregivers that emphasizes "chronicity" among those who use drugs. This model likens addiction to a lifelong disease, not unlike diabetes or asthma, which runs the risk of relapse without proper maintenance and care. In this characterization, addiction is outside the actor's control, and agency and power are relegated to those who work in treatment facilities or carceral settings. Further, the construction of an addiction as a "chronic, relapsing brain disorder" locates the problem in one's physiology rather than in the social world.

This definition of addiction produces an ideological link between drug use and other criminal activity: if you're addicted to drugs, you are understood as having a propensity for addiction to *other* bad things, too, which was reflected by interviewees like Sara, a twenty-two-year-old white woman, who explained that she was in prison because "I have an addictive personality." Similarly, Ingrid, a thirty-nine-year-old white woman, insisted that she is incarcerated because "I have a propensity for addiction." These narratives corroborate sociologist Allison McKim's research of addiction treatment centers, whereby women were taught that their chronic substance use and recidivism was the result of addictive personalities rather than external factors such as ineffective treatment programs, hyperpolicing, or the absence of other structural and interpersonal support systems.[24]

The biomedical model of addiction as disease shifts the governance paradigm from criminalizing to medicalizing substance use. As a result, the medicalization discourse perpetuates the same problems as the moral or criminal ones. In his ethnography of methamphetamine use in a rural US community, anthropologist William Garriott notes how doctors use the "chronic, recurring brain disease" model of addiction to explain individual propensities toward crime, thereby constructing groups as biologically predisposed to incarceration.[25]

Thus the model biologizes criminality—one is born an addict and a criminal rather than being constructed as one by those in power. This perspective is articulated by Missouri state senator Rob Schaaf, who once argued that when people die of a drug overdose, it "just removes them from the gene pool."[26] For Schaaf and others who share his perspective, people who use drugs are bad people with bad genetics and society would benefit from their removal or isolation. Interviewees' frequent references to themselves as addicts reflect an internalization of this perspective. They also reflect the internalization of a discourse of chronicity—of addiction and incarceration—and the normalization of individuals moving between different institutions of control.

"It's a Rat Factory": Biopower as Rehabilitation

The number of individuals incarcerated for drug offenses in the United States increased tenfold between 1980 and 2017, from 40,900 to 452,900. Almost half of all federal prisoners had been convicted of a drug offense, and nine times as many state prisoners were incarcerated on drug charges in 2017 as in 1980.[27] Today, prisoners spend considerably longer behind bars than they did forty years ago as a result of determinate sentencing, which, by the late 1990s, had been adopted by all fifty states. Judges were increasingly held to uniform sentencing guidelines, such as mandatory minimums and "truth in sentencing" policies that require that offenders not be released before 85 percent of their sentence has been served—guidelines that were supported by "tough on crime" conservatives and liberals fearful of discriminatory and arbitrary judgment.[28] The effects of these policies have been monumental: "Whereas in the past, first-time or low-level offenders might have been placed on probation instead of in prison, new sentencing laws imposed stricter punishments for a broad range of offenses. The chances of receiving a prison sentence following arrest increased by more than 50 percent as a result of determinate sentencing laws."[29] As of 2016, almost three-quarters of federal prisoners were convicted of an offense with a mandatory minimum penalty, under laws that require that a judge hand down a minimum prison sentence for certain charges. As a result, the average prison sentence was ninety-four months, more than four times the average prison sentence in 1986 (twenty-two months) and double the average sentence for drug offenders who were convicted of an offense that did not carry a mandatory minimum penalty (forty-two months).[30]

But another factor that may be contributing to increases in prison populations is the volume approach to surveillance, arrest, and imprisonment. During the 1980s, the United States witnessed a significant shift in approach to policing, particularly in regard to illicit substances. Adopting a volume approach to policing, the Reagan administration launched Operation Pipeline, a training program funded by the Drug Enforcement Administration that trained state police and highway patrol officers how to engage in high-volume traffic stops with the aim of searching vehicles and personal items for illicit substances. The program also provided real-time communication with other police departments and analytic support, to facilitate swift identification of individuals with records. The pipeline approach assumes that anyone might be a potential criminal and therefore should be interrogated. Rehabilitation programs increasingly operate in a similar fashion, training patients to surveil and police one another, allowing surveillance and potential punishment to be anywhere and everywhere. The assumption is the same: anyone with a documented record of illicit drug activity is a potential suspect of future illicit activity. And constructing participation in the surveillance system as an indicator of recovery allows such programs to enlist the labor of patients at no financial cost, thereby increasing the efficiency and expansiveness of the approach.

In theory, treatment should be the opposite of incarceration. While incarceration involves punishment, treatment should offer support. However, this assumes that the individuals in these programs are in need of intervention and that the treatment in fact provides support rather than harm. All our interviewees had participated in some form of inpatient or outpatient rehabilitation program; yet, the majority argued that the programs involved more punishment than support. For example, Grant, a fifty-three-year-old white man who has been arrested over one hundred times in his life, describes how the programs he attended "ain't nothing about drugs and alcohol." He describes how in each of his mandated programs, it was all about "behavior modification. Try to teach you how to act and whatever." From Grant's perspective, the programs should have "treated what was wrong with you. If dope caused it, you know, treat you for dope." Instead, "they want to teach you how to tell on somebody. It just don't work."

Like Grant, others argued that rehabilitation programs focused less on support and more upon enlisting their efforts in policing each other. Several brought up the fact that programs required patients to "rat" on one another or to file a "pull-up," which was a report on someone not engaging in "proper" behavior as outlined by the facility's code of conduct. Ronald, a fifty-six-year-old white man, argues that "the drug treatment program in prison requires me to tell on you and to write pull-ups on you. When people write pull-ups on you, you get a sanction. And pretty soon, you are spending more time bearing resentment and hatred than you are paying attention to your problem. It should be responsible telling. No. It's not responsible telling. All right? It's a rat factory. You're teaching people how to tell on one another." A number of respondents described how the imperative to police others bleeds outside of the program, effectively creating Jeremy Bentham's panopticon described by Michel Foucault in *Discipline and Punish*.[31] The successful panopticon convinces the prisoner that they are always being watched; in doing so, they monitor each other as well as themselves. This strategy may have originated in the prison, but it has extended outward as patients at treatment centers are taught how to "get clean" by becoming part of the carceral state; policing themselves and others has become a sign of sobriety and good citizenship. This strategy establishes users and nonusers as two distinct communities at war with one another.

Sobriety comes with moral superiority as well as policing power. That policing power is oriented outward, but also inward, often fracturing one's sense of self as patients are taught that part of them is bad, immoral, or manipulative and that the good part must monitor and control the bad part. Respondents who had participated in mandated treatment programs described them as "abusive" and "a waste of time." For example, Betsy describes the punitive discourse in treatment programs as "ridiculous. In there, they're very abusive. I'm not going to have somebody tear me down and tell me that I'm a piece of shit." She describes how in such diversion treatment programs, facilitators told her that she was "nothing, how I had never amounted to anything, and if I don't start doing this or doing that I'm never going to amount to anything. That's not the truth."

Yet the impact of such programs is serious. Individuals often internalize these messages and therefore struggle with the associated character assumptions, or the expectation of their recidivism or relapse. With systems of surveillance and policing established everywhere, those who need support the most may instead isolate themselves as a means of protection. Many people who use drugs do so because they feel isolated already. They are disconnected from the workforce, from neoliberal notions of productivity, and from their families and friends. Such policies and practices that inculcate paranoia and fear may only intensify these experiences and push individuals to greater substance use and greater isolation—a potentially lethal combination.

Prisons in the United States are overcrowded.[32] People are housed in unsafe conditions or in spaces that exceed capacity. This is partly attributable to the "revolving door" of the prison system, whereby individuals who have been incarcerated are more likely to be reincarcerated. As an illustration of such trends, over three-quarters of state offenders arrested on drug charges were rearrested within five years of their offense.[33] Rather than rethinking legislation that requires locking up so many people, government has increasingly extended surveillance and control outside of the prison to include electronic monitoring systems and mandated treatment programs, all of which is referred to as the "net widening" of the carceral system. Yet, as demonstrated by these accounts, this net widening exists within these programs as well, as patients are enlisted as additional eyes for prison guards, case workers, and law enforcement officers.

The individuals we spoke to had suffered considerable harms during their lives—some of them preceding medicalization and criminalization, others following. All those we spoke to became trapped in the contradictions of the health-care and carceral systems that simultaneously under- and overtreat conditions with pharmaceutical solutions and criminalize the consequences of that model of care. The prescription-to-prison pipeline is the result of a system that blames individuals rather than addressing the underlying social, political, and financial issues that directly contribute to the drug use in the first place. If we want to see different outcomes, we need to rethink the systems and society that produce them. In the conclusion, I explore structural, policy, and cultural shifts that may yield a more humane and just system.

CONCLUSIONS

WHEN MEDICINE BECOMES A DRUG

The fact that the United States consumes more opioids and psychotropics than any other nation and is also home to the largest prison population in the world is no mere coincidence. It reflects the intimate link between medicine and prisons as social institutions and how each one reinforces the power of the other. Both medicine and prisons are used to classify, control, and treat individuals who often lack the resources or power to protest. While prescription drugs have increasingly been replacing comprehensive mental health treatment, penalties for their nonmedical use have increased. That prescription drugs are increasingly treated as a panacea for social problems while also serving as a justification for criminalization is a serious issue as it allows both medicine and prisons to magnify and extend their power, often to the detriment of the already marginalized.

Despite the often noble intentions of those working in hospitals, psychiatrist offices, rehabilitation centers, or even prisons, these institutions have the ability to exacerbate and reentrench preexisting axes of inequality. Through systems of classification, diagnosis, intervention, and surveillance, medical subjects are disciplined via constant monitoring and measuring according to singular standards of physical and mental health as well as psychological and moral fitness. These standards are racialized, gendered, and classed in ways that result in worse health outcomes and higher rates of incarceration and premature death for marginalized individuals.

This book pushes us to interrogate how, when, and whom medicine or prisons serve, and for whom they produce or exacerbate existing problems. It asks us to interrogate why the United States has a declining life span, some of the greatest racial disparities in health, and one of the highest maternal childbirth mortality rates in the world, despite spending more on health care than any other nation. In a nation of plenty, the suffering of our poor and other underserved populations is a reflection of failed social policy and collective indifference to injustice.

The title of the book, *The Prescription-to-Prison Pipeline*, draws a parallel between the punitive disciplinary measures used in a highly stratified school system (e.g., suspension, expulsion) that are highly predictive of future incarceration; a War on Drugs tactical program that focuses on surveilling, searching, and arresting mass numbers of people under the pretext of protection; and the similar strategies of underresourcing and overpolicing certain groups who use prescription drugs. The connection is designed to make us reconsider under what conditions, and for whom, medicine is constructed as an unequivocal good, and how medicine is transformed into a drug in ways that justify surveillance and punishment of already marginalized individuals and groups.

Our contemporary legal and political systems protect those in power and punish those without. "Off-label" prescribing by physicians is legally protected, while nonmedical prescription drug use is criminally punished. Individuals who use substances face the brunt of the criminalization of nonmedical drug use, while manufacturers and physicians are rarely prosecuted.[1] Drug legislation pathologizes adaptive behaviors, such as taking substances to help focus at work, to manage trauma, to cope with physical and emotional demands of care work, or to find pleasure in an environment with few other sources of joy.

This conclusion begins with a call for a radical reform to our systems of both health care and law, with particular attention to how these reforms may dismantle systems of oppression. In doing so, it also issues a call to hold various stakeholders—including doctors, pharmaceutical companies, policy makers, and parents—accountable for their participation in a system that produces greater pain and incarceration and exacerbates inequality. However, remedying the situation needs to begin outside of medicine and the law. It needs to happen in the communities and environments where individuals experience pain in the first place. In a society stratified by race, class, gender, and a panoply of other factors, pain will continue to be stratified as well. While some of this stratification is produced at the hands of police officers, judges, doctors, or pharmaceutical companies, much of it is at the hands of policy makers deciding whether to grant the United States paid family leave, how to fund public schools and communities, and what kinds of unemployment benefits and support systems are available. This is purposely a much broader focus that implicates us all. The intention is to refocus attention away from individuals and substances and onto reforming the structures and policies that have both incentivized and criminalized nonmedical prescription drug use.

Despite its significant role, the pharmaceutical industry—and the health-care field more broadly—is not solely responsible for the medicalization or pharmaceuticalization of society. The pharmaceutical industry can accomplish its mission—the discovery, development, production, and marketing of drugs—only because it is supported by a large network of scientists, state regulators, hospitals, insurers, physicians, pharmacists, psychiatrists, prison workers, health social movements, and consumers. The pharmaceutical industry relies on (1) state and local lawmakers and politicians to regulate and oversee pharmaceutical products and set frameworks for their use, (2) physicians and pharmacists, who serve as gatekeepers for their products, (3) insurers, who pay the bill for these drugs, and (4) consumers, who drive demand.[2] But it also relies on a neoliberal economy in which individuals are responsible for their health and wealth, even when working and living conditions are incompatible with those efforts. Although the interests of this broader network of social actors do not always align with Big Pharma's goals, taken as a whole, this matrix of institutions, professions, and consumers determines which pharmaceuticals are produced and to whom they are available, leaving many to be under- or overmedicated as a consequence.

As the interviewees described in this book, those working low-wage jobs are more likely to incur injuries on the job and less likely to have access to health care or the time to appropriately take care of physical or mental health. Those raised in communities of simultaneous over- and underpolicing are the same people exposed to violence, trauma, and poverty, as their families have often been fractured by the carceral state: more than five million children in the United States have had a parent incarcerated, and half of all prisoners are parents.[3] Mothers are often provided prescription drugs before, during, or after childbirth but not provided adequate maternal leave, childcare, or a living wage.[4] As a consequence, it is often all but impossible to balance caretaking and breadwinning responsibilities. Partners are similarly not provided with parental leave in order to support their families. Employers need to be held accountable for making sure their laborers do not suffer physical or emotional hardship, but they also need to be supported to do so rather than being trapped in a race to the bottom, where low-wage jobs are increasingly stripped of all protections and benefits, while high-salary jobs experience the inverse. A living wage that makes it possible to support a family and participate in that family is a crucial step in this process that requires federal, state, and local interventions. Finally, we need to look at the disproportionate amount of funding we devote to police to address social problems, as opposed to investing in health care, education, and treatment that might prevent—rather than produce or exacerbate—suffering.

In her book *Body and Soul: The Black Panther Party and the Fight against Medical Discrimination*, sociologist Alondra Nelson traces the Black Panther Party's efforts to democratize health care through their "social health" approach. Nelson argues that this "elastic" frame drew connections between the health of "the individual, corporeal body to the body politic in such a way that therapeutic matters were inextricably articulated to social justice ones."[5] She explains how, "as a praxis, social health linked medical services to a program of societal transformation. The Panthers' clinics, for example, were imagined as sites of social change where preventive medicine was dispensed alongside both extramedical services (e.g., food banks and employment assistance) and ideology via the Party's political education (PE) classes" that provided a "unique critical discourse of citizenship and health rights."[6] This is a model that has influenced contemporary health-care debates and changes, including the public health-care option established by the Obama administration and the inclusion of cultural diversity and sociology education in health-care fields so that practitioners learn to communicate effectively and with respect to individuals from different backgrounds. Establishing more robust procedures for evaluating informed consent and protecting vulnerable populations from coercive treatment or research are other positive changes that can be traced to the Black Panther Party's efforts. And yet, the notion of "social health" has still not been fully realized in the United States, and this is essential to resolving these ecological issues.

Access to quality health care and mental health care is necessary as both a preventive measure and a safety net to catch those who may be overcome by life's hardships. In our current neoliberal model, which lacks necessary supports, taking care of yourself and your family is entirely the responsibility of the individual. In such a world, everyone runs the risk of bad medical luck, where an ailment can run up medical bills. However, those with greater economic, social, or cultural capital are protected from the associated consequences of that bad luck, which include the increased likelihood of experiencing unemployment, homelessness, and incarceration. Historically, only those with greater resources have had access to consistent medical care. Today, that translates into access to preventive medicine and trusting relationships with primary care doctors. Those without resources in the United States receive the bulk of their care in emergency rooms or in exchanges with pharmacists. Given this disparity, it would be worthwhile to provide greater training and support to health-care workers such as pharmacists, social workers, school counselors, and nurses. Sociologist Liz Chiarello suggests the United States ought to make greater use of pharmacists and pharmacies as they are often on the front lines of dealing with health issues, including substance dependence. While more intensive treatment would be beneficial, so would easily accessible, affordable, and regular contact with health-care professionals, which can often be provided by trained pharmacists and other frontline health workers such as those working in needle exchanges and vaccination clinics as well as school nurses, counselors, and workplace health workers.[7] Further collaboration between the siloed fields of criminal justice, public health, and medical practitioners could bring about important changes in how nonmedical prescription drug use is treated, but also in understanding what factors contribute to its emergence.[8]

People in each of these professions should receive training on how and when to use buprenorphine and methadone—medications approved by the FDA to treat opioid use disorder—effectively. Given the variability in needs, treatments should be individually tailored to individuals. While some would benefit from medication-assisted therapy, others would benefit from greater psychosocial support. Some need more structure, others need less. People need treatment that is complementary to their needs rather than a "one size fits all" model.

Our current health-care system is often program- rather than patient-centered, which increases the failure rates of such programs. This is as much true for the carceral system as it is for rehabilitation and treatment programs. If a methadone clinic opens at 8:00 a.m., but a person's work shift starts at 7:00 a.m., then they have to choose between treatment and holding down a job. Similarly, curfew may begin at 8:00 p.m., but without reliable transportation and with a work shift that ends at 7:00 p.m. across town, an individual may be flagged as violating conditions of parole despite their best efforts to get home in time. We should be aiding people to better understand their bodies and their needs rather than surveilling and punishing them for a bus running late, holding down a job, or using prescriptions in ways that diverge from doctor's orders.

Providers should be trained to develop empathy for patients by listening to their stories with the goal of understanding rather than fixing. This involves abandoning the notion of a "gold standard" that applies across all groups for a model that seeks to adapt to individual needs. Treatment centers that utilize psychotherapeutic techniques—focusing on the person and using talk therapy to understand past trauma and social issues—were found more effective by our respondents, confirming previous research,[9] and should be implemented and covered more broadly by our health-care system, particularly for the most disadvantaged. But these programs must extend beyond the walls of treatment facilities into the broader social environments that produced the pain in the first place. Above all else, they should be decoupled from a criminal legal system that only produces more harm, inequality, and pain.

Communities should have access to long-term and sustainable harm reduction initiatives, including medically assisted treatment programs such as supervised injection facilities, methadone clinics, buprenorphine and naloxone detox, and syringe access programs. Currently, many of these, such as naloxone—a life-saving medication—require a doctor's prescription and therefore are difficult to obtain. They should be available over the counter and in all public buildings, similar to fire extinguishers.

Patients who arrive in the emergency room in withdrawal should receive medication and support rather than morally infused forced sobriety. Withholding medication often runs counter to medical advice and increases the likelihood of death upon discharge. Although there are serious risks with combining buprenorphine or methadone with benzodiazepines or other central nervous system depressants, abruptly halting someone's medication or discharging them from the hospital setting can have deleterious effects.[10]

Denying individuals access to treatment is unethical. As an example, there are currently three drugs available on the US market to treat opioid dependence and overdose that have been found to be effective: methadone, buprenorphine, and naltrexone. Methadone and buprenorphine are partial agonists, meaning they stimulate the same part of the brain as other opioids and can produce euphoric sensations similar to more potent narcotics. However, they are much less potent than the most commonly used opioids, providing individuals with the ability to manage withdrawal symptoms and lessening cravings over time while dramatically reducing the risk of overdose. Critics of these substances argue that they merely replace one drug with another and that they run the risk of diversion. In contrast to methadone and buprenorphine, naltrexone is an antiagonist, meaning that it does not have addictive properties and is not an opioid. One cannot overdose from using naltrexone, and it does not run the risk of diversion. For these reasons, some have pushed for it to be the only medically assisted treatment option. However, studies find that *only* methadone and buprenorphine are effective at reducing risk of opioid overdose or serious opioid-related acute care; naltrexone is not.[11] Despite this fact, it often remains the only publicly funded option, contributing to the 500,000 deaths caused by drug overdose since the turn of the century.[12]

We have the ability to end the gridlock between pain management and addiction prevention initiatives, but only if we exhaust all available options and resources and build trust between patients and care providers. People need access to culturally sensitive health care and mental health support. Both physical and economic access is tantamount.

Health care should be woven into the fabric of our society. A living wage is health care. Secure, well-compensated, safe jobs are health care. Protection from violence is health care. Police who work with and serve every community are health care. Family, child, and elder support are health care. Dismantling racist, sexist, homophobic, and xenophobic systems of exclusion is health care. Rehabilitation treatment and support services are health care. Prison abolition is health care. Medicine is one part of health care, but ideally, a very small part. The rest are parts of systems that care for our health: health *care*. With proper preventive public health measures, medicine would be merely one small part of the system.

Deconstructing the Punitive Model

Doctors and pharmaceutical companies are rarely held responsible for their role in the overprescription of psychotropics and opioids, and neither are the regulatory bodies that oversee them. Insisting that relapse and recidivism are the norm and the fault of the individual's "chronic, relapsing brain disorder" rather than ineffective treatment or reintegration support system is a strategy for shirking responsibility and distracting focus from the conditions that contribute to substance use in the first place. However, criminalizing and punishing more individuals and entities is not going to solve these problems. In fact, it may simply create new ones.

From April 2020 to April 2021, more than 100,000 people died of a drug overdose in the United States. This was the first time that drug-related deaths had reached over six figures in a twelve-month period. Exacerbated by the COVID-19 pandemic and its effects, drug overdose and dependence increased across the board. While these numbers increased in response to stressors such as financial insecurity, loss of loved ones, and social isolation, they also likely increased as a result of shuttered methadone and needle exchange clinics and the stoppage of other harm reduction initiatives that help prevent such outcomes. The COVID-19 pandemic stripped away some of the most effective strategies for mitigating substance issues: social support, consistent health care, and social welfare programs. What was left was the punitive model that exacerbates rather than ameliorates these issues.

While drug overdose and dependence are significant, unresolved problems in the United States, our approaches to combating them only exacerbate their effects. People in recovery should have access to mutual support networks, stable recovery housing, and employment and mental health-care services, but so should the average person. Individuals should not have to wear a diagnostic or criminal label in order to be granted access to lifesaving care and support.[13] Programs that require participants to police one another or use methods such as solitary confinement only exacerbate the isolating and punitive effects of the carceral system, intensifying mental health issues in the process. Many of the most effective harm reduction strategies have been banned or underfunded by governments that seek to maintain these tenuous boundaries between medical use and abuse, licit and illicit substances. The very language of "harm reduction" itself implies that certain substances are uniformly harmful rather than beneficial in certain contexts.

These politically motivated moral boundaries are why the bulk of treatment facilities are part of the carceral state and offer only paltry care: both "addicts" and "criminals" are treated as second-class citizens, and treatment often resembles punishment more than rehabilitation or support. Once individuals leave prison or rehabilitation centers, many struggle to find employment and housing, to attend school, or to meet other basic human needs. As sociologist Devah Pager argues, many assume that "the kinds of people who wind up in prison don't really want to work, or don't have sufficient skills to find a job" without considering that "the experience of prison changes inmates in ways that make them less suited for the formal labor market," or that "the stigma of incarceration imposes barriers to finding employment."[14] Similarly, the methods by which substance use is treated in the United States create and exacerbate the very issues that they purport to solve by forcing people to adopt labels of addicts and criminals and navigate the structural barriers that emerge in response.

As millions of people in the United States suffer the consequences of overprescription and dependence in conjunction with inadequate health care and mental health support, many state lawmakers have sought to deal with these problems through the criminal justice system, despite empirical evidence that greater criminalization of drugs or "tough on crime" approaches, such as mandatory minimum sentences for drug offenses, are not effective in curbing drug use or abuse. It was for this reason that Eric Holder, the attorney general under President Barack Obama, instructed prosecutors to "refine our charging policy regarding mandatory minimums for certain nonviolent, low-level, drug offenders," given that "long sentences for low-level, non-violent drug offenses do not promote public safety, deterrence, or rehabilitation." However, President Donald

Trump rescinded these instructions once he came to office. Specifically, Attorney General Jeff Sessions encouraged prosecutors to "charge and pursue the most serious, readily provable offense" even against low-level, nonviolent drug offenders.[15] State lawmakers followed suit. At least sixteen states added "tough on crime" legislation purposely targeting opioids after 2016 despite the fact that punitive "tough on crime" initiatives have had no bearing on drug prices or drug use.[16]

The spike in incarceration rates in the United States over the last forty years is not the result of increasing rates in violence or individual-inflicted harm. Instead, it reflects shifts in legislation that have transformed noncriminal activity into criminal activity. Almost half of all people serving time in federal prisons have been convicted of a drug offense. Nine times as many state prisoners were incarcerated on drug charges in 2017 than in 1980.[17]

While the decriminalization of drug use would be a good place to start in deconstructing the punitive penal system, the majority of those who end up incarcerated do so as a result of community supervision infractions: breaking the terms associated with probation, parole, or pretrial supervision. Such "technical violations" include breaking curfew or failing to pay unaffordable supervision fees. Community supervision programs stigmatize people through labels and perpetual surveillance systems that expect reoffending and recidivism rather than reintegration. While probation could be used to reduce mass incarceration, it presently serves as a form of "net widening," entrenching more people in the system and in many cases contributing to increased—rather than decreased—rates of incarceration.[18]

The disenfranchisement of the formerly incarcerated contributes to a structural design that all but ensures recidivism. As legal scholar Michelle Alexander argues, "Once a person is labeled a felon, he or she is ushered into a parallel universe in which discrimination, stigma, and exclusion are perfectly legal, and privileges of citizenship such as voting and jury service are off-limits." As a result, "it does not matter whether you have actually spent time in prison; your second-class citizenship begins the moment you are branded a felon."[19] This is increasingly true for those who have been branded an "addict." Individuals receive worse medical care and are often treated with mistrust, which causes vital relationships to deteriorate. We should move away from a classificatory system that relies upon reductive labels. In relying on such classificatory systems, we resort to hyperstandardization of care that often only exacerbates conditions, particularly among the already underserved and hypersurveilled.

Both substance use and its treatment have become central to carceral power. As many others have chronicled, treatment has taken a coercive and punitive turn, adhering to the same principles of carceral punishment.[20] People should not have to be criminalized in order to gain access to treatment, and those who receive treatment should be able to do so with respect and a holistic approach intended to understand individuals as people rather than as "addicts," "felons," or "abusers." Treatment should also not be limited to inpatient rehabilitation centers, which come with the expectation that a short stay will transform one's life. Instead, treatment and prevention should be integrated into society at every level—including better access to health care, more comprehensive insurance coverage, alternative forms of therapy, and robust harm reduction initiatives. Even more broadly, a living wage, affordable housing, free and quality education at all levels, affordable and accessible childcare, job training, and other economic and social policies could dramatically reduce problematic substance use by addressing its root causes.

The War on Drugs is not over. It is also not new. The United States has had a storied history with drug regulation, and the convergence between the prohibition of different substances and the populations who were associated with those substances can help us better understand what is actually at stake in drug regulation: the control, disenfranchisement, and abuse of racialized populations. While drug regulation policies are often presented as an effort to protect individuals or communities from harm, research has indicated that many who use mind-altering substances are those who are trying to escape harm in the first place. If the issue were truly about the health and well-being of these individuals and communities, then the trillions of dollars funneled into the War on Drugs would be diverted to housing, health care, childcare, and effective mental health, substance abuse, and trauma counseling.[21] This has been a resounding argument made by the "defund the police" and prison abolitionist movements that advocate for the redirection of resources away from policing and prisons toward institutions that prevent rather than produce pain.

After people receive treatment or are released from institutionalized settings such as rehabilitation centers or prisons, they are often left on their own, without assistance, as they struggle to find employment, housing, and a community to support them in staying clean. Therefore, it is important for policy initiatives to focus on community and structural support, and not just treating individuals once they have relapsed. Those who have been incarcerated find an entire world closed off to them as they are barred from housing, food, and financial assistance in the form of scholarships, loans, and public subsidy programs, as well as being legally discriminated against in the job market as applicants are often required to disclose their criminal background on job applications. Prison reformists have argued in favor of eliminating such restrictions on employment, housing, education, and other social services. However, the stigma of criminal records and the associated discrimination against those who have them are unlikely to disappear overnight even with policy reform. Hence, prison abolitionists question whether there should be prisons at all.[22] They push us to question whether the prison system accomplishes what it purports to—increasing safety and reforming offenders—or whether it seeks to exploit and harm already marginalized populations. If the latter is the case, we must reconsider whether this form of criminal justice accomplishes any justice at all.

The prison industrial complex thrives in a neoliberal, capitalist context that seeks to scale back welfare policies and expand the debt economy while simultaneously promulgating racialized criminal figures such as the "superpredator" or the drug dealer to justify the disinvestment in these communities and explain why some groups fare worse than others. These processes are exacerbated by a net widening of the prison system into what Jackie Wang calls a "carceral continuum" of juvenile detention, probation, increasing fees and fines associated with court appearances, bail, and the individual burden of paying for surveillance technologies associated with cybernetic governance.[23]

The prison industrial complex is designed to disenfranchise, stigmatize, and set people back so they are *more* likely to recidivate rather than less. People come out of the prison system worse off than they were before—financially, emotionally, socially, and psychologically—which is the precise intent of a punitive model that seeks to punish and stigmatize rather than rehabilitate or prevent recidivism. Recidivism is often treated as a bug in need of resolution in the current carceral system, when the truth is the recidivism is a fundamental part of this model. Restorative and transformative justice models offer alternatives to the punitive system by seeking to heal people and their trauma and provide consequences that may result in positive transformations for all involved.

The goal of a "justice" system should be to meet the needs of those who suffered harm, those who caused harm, and the affected communities. This stands in contrast to our current model, which focuses on individual punishment and too often results in negative consequences for all three entities through reverberating downstream effects.

Many crimes that are punished by the US criminal legal system do not harm anyone. If the intention of the system is to reduce harm, then we must reconsider what is criminalized and how the system seeks to remedy that harm. The goal is decriminalization, but not creating a system without consequences or justice. Instead, it pushes us to interrogate what true "justice" looks like and whether the current criminal "justice" system approximates that.

The Racialization Project of Prescription Drug Use

The opioid crisis identifies a substance as the source of social problems. However, these social problems exist even without these stimulating factors. Unemployment, poverty, health inequities, trauma, abuse, racism, sexism, homophobia, and xenophobia are serious issues that structure social life in the absence of pandemics and epidemics. They are endemic to our society. But they are not distributed evenly. In sociologist Celeste Watkins-Hayes's terms, many of these issues brought to our attention via "the opioid crisis" are actually "injuries of inequality—big and small wounds to personal, familial, and community well-being [that] represent the mental, physical, and social toll of acute inequity."[24] They have impacted economically and socially marginalized populations for a long time yet have only recently been brought to national attention as they began to impact more advantaged groups, such as white or economically secure populations. The shift away from entirely punitive models for addressing drug use to more rehabilitative approaches also came about only once those who were using and incarcerated for substance use became increasingly white and middle class. This is a departure from the racist history of incarceration in the United States, particularly tied to the War on Drugs. Today, the numerical majority of those who overdose from opioids are white.[25]

This book chronicles a recent phenomenon—the criminalization of non-medical use of prescription drugs. However, neither the criminalization of substance use nor the use of mind-altering substances to treat pain is a novel feature of US society. The power to classify certain behaviors or substances as legitimate and safe and others as criminal and risky has a long history, rooted in racial capitalism. This book chronicles how even the classifications of "medicine" and "drug" are conditional, based on who is using the substance, from whom it was obtained, and who profits from its use. In this moral—and financial—economy, the meanings of substance use are amorphous, often shifting to uphold particular structures of power.

In her book *The New Jim Crow*, legal scholar and civil rights activist Michelle Alexander chronicles how prisons have become "racemaking institutions." Specifically, Alexander traces how drug legislation in the United States has produced the disproportionate incarceration of people of color, particularly Black men, but also how discrimination against people with a criminal record legalizes (and legitimizes) racial discrimination. While it is technically illegal to discriminate against someone on the basis of one's skin tone, it is not illegal to discriminate on the basis of one's criminal record. In this way, Alexander argues, people who become entangled in the criminal legal system are "made

Black" and thereby justifiably discriminated against. She points out that some white people are also incarcerated on drug charges but that they are not the intended targets of the racialized caste system produced by the New Jim Crow.[26]

This is most clearly evident in the fact that white people who are criminalized continue to reap the privileges of their whiteness. Drug courts and treatment facilities were implemented as a humanistic approach to rehabilitation and to keep people out of prison. However, the beneficiaries of this tiered system remain disproportionately white, as Black and Latinx individuals are more likely to be sent to prison rather than to rehab.[27] In contrast to the Black individuals who used crack in the 1980s, white opioid users are often portrayed as victims. This reflects a double standard in drug legislation and portrayal whereby white people have historically been on the classifying end of the racialization project, constructing whiteness as innocent and Blackness as guilty. And yet, white people are serving time for their substance use more often. They accumulate criminal records that result in being barred from housing, employment, education, and financial assistance programs reserved for those without a criminal record. In Alexander's terms, they are increasingly "made Black" in legal terms, though they still retain their white privilege in terms of their deservingness and sympathy. To be clear: the goal here is not to villainize or punish these white individuals *more*, but rather to interrogate why their nonwhite counterparts are not extended the same empathy and compassion.

Approaches to these issues should be grounded in compassion and the desire to understand rather than in punishment and fear. Holding pharmaceutical companies, doctors, and legislators accountable for the consequences of manufacturing, prescribing, and regulating prescription drugs is an important step in transformative justice. However, the goal should not be to increase criminalization by punishing producers and prescribers rather than users. Instead, the goal should be to collectively reassess what our moral and social obligations are to one another: If we have the right to live and to be free of physical, psychological, and emotional pain, how might we go about securing those associated rights and protections in this country? Prioritizing profit over personhood is one way that our current system is designed to promote harm and pain of all kinds. As a result, pain is caused before, during, and after the criminalization process. Pharmaceuticals only exacerbate this process by protecting doctors and companies from impunity as patients and prisoners are further harmed.

If prescription drugs that are pharmacologically similar to street drugs are legal and covered by health insurance, then we must reconsider why other substances are prohibited. Does prohibition really protect individuals from harm, or does the prohibition only create further harms as individuals are policed, punished, incarcerated, and disenfranchised for their use? This punitive model has not resulted in reduced substance use or associated negative outcomes but rather has ushered in new problems, many of which are concentrated in already marginalized communities. The legalization of drugs—rather than mere decriminalization—would be a way to undo these new harms and develop the infrastructure for helping rather than punishing people who often started using drugs as a means of coping with other hardship and pain.

As noted at the beginning of this book, nonmedical prescription drug use is predicated on a number of contradictions: how a licit substance is made illicit, but only in certain contexts or for certain individuals. But perhaps the greatest contradiction is how nonmedical prescription drug use has inverted the classic racist framing of substance use in this country and its associated criminalization. The opioid epidemic has been framed differently than the War on Drugs precisely because historically, affluent white individuals had greater access to prescription drugs. This population has been framed as well-intentioned consumers and patients rather than hedonistic criminals. It is this framework and story that have spurred the investment in treatment centers and universal health care, the increasing use of drug courts, and the call to decriminalize or even legalize substance use. While some of these are positive developments, it is important to draw attention to the fact that this legal, political, and cultural shift is the product of a racialization project constructing opioids and other pharmaceuticals as fundamentally different from illicit substances. The fact that the call for reform came only when drug legislation began to impact white, middle-class families in negative ways makes evident how the system has always been designed to protect some groups and disenfranchise others. While change is long overdue, as these changes are implemented, it is important to consider how they will uphold or dismantle the underlying systems of racism, classism, and sexism.

Rethinking Pain

The pain that interviewees experienced was the result of structural inequality: poverty, racism, sexism, and exposure to violence and trauma, issues that ought not fall exclusively under the purview of the medical establishment. These are economic and political issues that ought to be remedied by broader legislation that secures housing, employment, and protection against violence rather than medications to numb the symptoms of such inequality. Yet medications were prescribed for trauma and abuse, much like they were prescribed for physical pain incurred from injury and violence. Therefore, the solutions occur at the individual, corporal level rather than the collective, ideological, or infrastructural one, even though this results in treatment of the symptoms rather than the underlying causes that may be more complex and contextual than as depicted by medical or scientific literature. As doctors and judges underestimate the economic, political, and social (racialized, gendered, sexualized) dimensions of pain, their solutions will continue to focus on the body and the brain, ignoring the environments in which bodies and brains are nourished and grow or wither and die.

Poverty and the associated pains of oppression are the fundamental cause (or causes) of opiate and other drug use. The opposite is also true: social welfare programs that provide access to affordable and safe housing, quality education, job training and employment opportunities, healthy and accessible food, and exhaustive health care are correlated with greater education and employment outcomes, as well as lower rates of incarceration and child separation within communities.[28] In the absence of these services at a national level, we continue to live through a public health crisis that is only exacerbated by pharmaceutical solutions.

Incarcerated people are often blamed for making "bad choices" that resulted in drug dependency, and they are regularly told that their social marginalization is the result of poor decisions rather than preceding structural inequities. Rather than focusing on poverty or social dislocation as sources of drug use or incarceration, many penal institutions flip the script and promote the same popular discourse that exists outside of prison walls: bad choices and bad actors are responsible for ending up in bad environments. The women in sociologist Lynne Haney's 2010 study of community-based prisons were similar to many of our interviewees. As Haney describes, "Despite these women's many differences, most of their problems had social roots: the women all faced poverty and restricted access to public support; they all came from neighborhoods decimated by abandonment and neglect; and they all struggled to keep their familial bonds intact despite histories of absence and abuse. It took an enormous amount out of these women to survive—materially, physically, and emotionally—in the communities they came from and would soon return to."[29] Despite these fraught histories, prison guards, social workers, doctors, and judges alike blame offenders for making bad choices rather than being critical of the social policies that cause greater harm and trauma for certain groups of people or of the overreliance on the carceral system to manage social problems.

People use drugs when they are in pain. However, environments that provide emotional, social, and financial support and intellectual stimulation have been linked to less drug use since these factors mitigate such pain. In the classic study used to justify abstinence-only, punitive drug policies, a rat is placed in a bare cage with a bottle of water and a bottle of sweetened morphine. Over time, the rat is drawn to the pleasure-inducing morphine, using it in greater quantities until it eventually overdoses and dies. This study has been used as a justification for outlawing drugs such as heroin and cocaine, arguing that the drugs themselves are so addictive that they will necessarily result in overdose and death. However, these studies, like most others, were all conducted in bare cages, where rats were isolated and exposed to surveillance—two factors that produce anxiety and distress for rats (and humans, too, as it turns out).

In 1981, a Canadian psychologist, Bruce Alexander, and his colleagues offered a rebuttal to this argument through their own research. In a project called "Rat Park," Alexander sought to understand how rats would use heroin-laced water when placed in a larger cage, with items desirable to rodents, such as training wheels, toys, food, and water, in addition to sexually receptive mates. In these environments, while some rats would use heroin intermittently, most preferred the plain water. This was true even when the heroin-laced water was sweetened like candy to be intensely desirable or when rats were given large doses of drugs for two weeks before so that they were experiencing intense withdrawal symptoms.[30] It was only those rats placed in cramped, isolated quarters that continued to use the drugs. The others abstained or used in moderation. Other research with prairie voles has found that they demonstrate less interest in amphetamines when in a bonded relationship than when single.[31]

This research demonstrates that individuals with socially and intellectually stimulating environments and close, loving relationships are less likely to use drugs, especially to use them to the point of dependence or overdose. It challenges the notion that it is the pharmacological properties of substances or one's genetic propensity for addiction that leads to substance use or "abuse." Instead, it suggests that the absence of intellectual stimulation, social connection, or employment opportunities to activate and motivate ambition is responsible for negative outcomes. If someone is left alone all day and night, without social contact or affection, quality education, employment, or social mobility, but has access to drugs, then those drugs suddenly become very appealing. They make the person using the drug feel good, or at least OK, for a few hours. They are even more appealing if authorized by a medical authority as they are considered healthy and legitimate, especially if "prescribed by my doctor."

Some of us live in "Rat Park" and others live in the bare cage—in prison cells or in underfunded communities. In an experimental setting, we can easily see these impacts, but the extensive research on the social determinants of health makes all too clear the same conclusion: those who are supported will do well, and those who are not will suffer. Pathologizing adaptive behaviors such as taking substances to hold down jobs, to stay safe on the streets at night, or to experience pleasure in environments that provide very little only makes life more painful and prescription drugs more palatable. If the goal is the opposite, then it seems obvious that we focus on initiatives such as housing first, job training and quality public education, treatment on demand, and other harm reduction programs. In the end, it is all about the reckoning and reconceptualization of central questions. What is a medicine, and what is a drug? What produces harm in our society, and what ameliorates it? By asking and answering these questions truthfully, we can envision a new world.

Much of the criminal justice system relies on storytelling—the ability of a prosecutor or a defendant to tell a convincing story using and constructing evidence in particular ways. The jury and the judge must be convinced to make a decision one way or another. This book is grounded in stories—of the individuals who shared their personal experiences as well as the story of racialized drug legislation in the United States—culminating in a new story. The goal of that story is to convince important stakeholders—lawyers, judges, policy makers, pharmacists, pharmaceutical companies, and people who use substances, as well as the general population—that the current approaches to nonmedical prescription drug use are not effective and are ultimately producing greater harms. Those closest to the problem are often closest to the solutions; therefore, we must be willing to listen and take their stories very seriously. We must be willing to transform systems in accordance with their stories. We must be willing to speak truth to power.

APPENDIX

METHODOLOGICAL NOTE

Institutional review boards (IRBs) at each university set guidelines for conducting research on human populations. Before researchers begin to collect data, talk to people, or send out surveys, each project must be reviewed by a panel of fellow researchers at the institution to make sure that the research poses no undue harm to the population being studied and, even further, that the research is not exploiting particularly vulnerable populations. There are a number of protected categories of persons that are deemed particularly vulnerable: children or persons under eighteen years of age, people who are developmentally disabled, pregnant women, and incarcerated persons. Some of these groups are considered vulnerable because they are unable to freely give consent, they may not fully understand the risks associated with participating, or they may feel pressured to consent if they are housed in an institutionalized setting. The use of coercion in research is strictly forbidden. However, what constitutes coercion is often more challenging to discern than one might assume. It is up to the researcher and the IRB to evaluate each study.

Prior to accepting my current appointment as an assistant professor at the University of Missouri–Kansas City, I worked for the Census Bureau in the Center for Survey Measurement. This is a center where we developed and pretested many of the questions that appear in national surveys. I conducted hundreds of these interviews while I was working at the Census. There, the policy was always to pay respondents a forty-dollar incentive to compensate for their transportation and time spent participating in the interview. For focus groups that lasted one and a half to two hours, we paid participants seventy-five dollars. During one of our collaborative projects with the Office of Management and Budget (OMB) where we were exploring trust in statistical agencies, we specifically sought out unhoused respondents as members of our study. Unhoused people are chronically undercounted, and their needs are underreported, in part because they are often mistrustful of surveyors and other representatives of government power. Halfway through this research, we were halted by OMB, which had found out that we were paying our respondents the standard forty or seventy-five dollars for their participation. They argued that such large sums of money were considered to be coercive when given to a respondent with unstable housing or employment. While these amounts were standard and used widely across all branches of the United States government, these researchers were lobbying for an exception to be made when interviewing respondents under a particular income threshold (though what exactly constituted such a threshold was never defined). My colleagues and I fought back, arguing that paying some people less than others for the same labor constitutes a breach of ethics. It was also discriminatory on the basis of one's housing or income status. In such a scenario, we wrestled with the tension between coercion and equality. If the labor on the interview is the same—one or two hours' worth of time—then what is the justification for paying some populations forty dollars per hour and another only twenty dollars per hour? Considering that many of our housed respondents were between jobs or similarly motivated to participate because they needed the extra money, were any of those interviews free from coercion? Who agrees to participate in research, and who has the luxury to decline? These questions are much thornier than they may appear on the surface.

The IRB at the University of Missouri–Kansas City approved criminologist Jennifer Owens's and my proposal to survey and interview incarcerated people about their nonmedical prescription drug use. We were motivated to speak to incarcerated people given that they are not included in nationally representative surveys and their stories offer unique details that are not systematically captured in studies of other noninstitutionalized populations. But even further, we were interested in the relationship between nonmedical prescription drugs and illicit substances, as well as how nonmedically using prescription drugs contributed to their incarceration. Have prescription drugs been criminalized for some populations rather than others? And if so, what contributes to disproportionate policing?

While the UMKC IRB approved our study and we went forward with the surveys and interviews with these incarcerated people, I still struggle with the question of whether this research was coercive or exploitive. Each of our survey respondents was compensated five dollars for completing the two-page survey, and those who participated in the interviews were paid twenty dollars. These amounts of money are considerable in prison; in Missouri, prisoners are paid between five cents and $1.25 per hour for their labor while locked up. The national average is between fourteen cents and $1.41 per hour.[1] While the United States takes some measures to protect nonincarcerated persons from exploitive work through the establishment of wage minimums and overtime pay criteria, incarcerated people are not protected by those laws. Therefore, their earning potential while locked up is minimal. And given their inability to vote while in prison—and, for many felons, indefinitely after they are released—such policies are unlikely to change. In many ways, incarcerated people are rendered invisible—excluded from nationally representative research; barred from voting and from receiving financial assistance for education or housing; and unable to earn, consume, or produce as the nonincarcerated do. Paying twenty dollars or even five dollars is substantial, but is it fair? Is it coercive? These are all questions that qualitative researchers must grapple with in conducting research, particularly upon vulnerable populations. In a similar vein, we might ask: Is the military coercive? Is it exploitive? Do those people who choose to serve and risk their lives on behalf of their nation freely choose to do so? Or are they motivated by educational loans or paychecks that could support their families in the absence of other educational or occupational opportunities?

It is with all these questions in mind that I participated in this data collection and research. I continue to think of these questions as I write up my findings. In early 2019, I attended a panel at the Sociologists for Women in Society Winter Conference entitled Community Engagement and Scholar Activism. During this presentation, panelists discussed the duty that we have as researchers to listen to the communities that we serve and ask them what needs to be done. As academic researchers, they encouraged us to garner the trust of those we work with by demonstrating that we were committed to their cause. If they choose to include us, to open up to us, it is our imperative to use our access, our institutional resources, and our publication outlets in order to promote changes that benefit these communities. Listening to the inspiring work being conducted by these panelists was a reminder of my commitment as a scholar-activist to do something with the resources—and the privilege as a nonincarcerated, white, highly educated person—at my disposal.

The individuals we surveyed and interviewed do not have a voice. In this book, I aim to tell their stories. While I would have preferred to do this from a participatory research framework, I did not have the luxury of completing follow-up interviews or engaging in such a collaborative approach. This was the result of the many-layered guarantees established to protect our respondents' confidentiality and privacy. Specifically, Dr. Owens and I lobbied the IRB to allow us to use a waiver of documentation of consent rather than a traditional consent form that requires respondents to sign their names and be linked to the study. Instead, participants consented to participation in the research by reading the form and consenting to the interviewer. We also procured a certificate of confidentiality from the National Institute on Drug Abuse (DA-15-017) that protected our data from being subpoenaed by law enforcement officials during the periods between collecting the surveys and inputting the data in nonidentifiable terms and between the interviews and the transcription and disidentification of those conversations. To protect their identities, our data were disidentified and anonymized within days after data collection, so it was impossible to track down individuals and have them review the manuscript prior to publication. As a result of those protections, we could not identify our own respondents after the interviews even if we had so desired.

We did ask the people we interviewed about their recommendations for state policies and for our research, and I used these to guide part of the conclusion. Additionally, we made it very clear that they need not answer any question that made them uncomfortable. It was not our intention to pry information or to coerce information out of their narratives. We asked them to disidentify their own stories where possible—not use names or specific identifiable locations. We then completed another round of disidentification during the transcription process as we edited the transcripts. Our ultimate goal was to protect our respondents as our commitment to them and their causes was the heart of this research.

To recruit interview participants, Dr. Owens and I sent out 510 surveys to a random sample of prisoners at men's and women's correctional facilities in Missouri.[2] Of the 240 women who received surveys, 168 responded, yielding a 70 percent response rate. Of the 234 men who received surveys, 114 responded, yielding a 49 percent response rate. The survey asked detailed questions about frequency, conceptualization, and variety of Rx drug use, as well as detailed questions pertaining to how and when they began using and what were some of the ways they went about obtaining these drugs. The people who provided their name and ID number were given a five-dollar incentive and were eligible for the second part of the study: the qualitative interviews with nonmedical Rx drug users. It is this second portion that is the focus of this book.

The eighty people asked to participate in the interviews were purposively sampled from a survey based upon frequency and variety of Rx drug use, actuation behaviors, and level of "entrenchment" in the Rx drug scene (by virtue of dealing Rx drugs or participating in multiple avenues of actuation) prior to incarceration, because we believed those who were most entrenched would have the most to say on the subject. Surveys were collected on a Monday, and interviews commenced the following day. Interviews were completed in each prison over the course of two weeks. The interviews lasted, on average, forty minutes.

Each participant was provided with a detailed written description of the study, time to ask questions, and the opportunity to consent or decline participation. Interviews were conducted in private staff offices with closed doors so that only the principal investigators—Michelle Smirnova and Jennifer Owens—were able to hear their responses. Only two of the forty-two women asked to participate opted out, and only one of the forty-one men did. We informed all participants that their responses would be kept in confidence. In all our research, we use pseudonyms, and all identifiable information is omitted or changed.

Demographic information of the interview participants is included in table A.1. Of note is the racial and age composition of our samples. Of the women surveyed, 85.7 percent identified as white, as did over 90 percent of women who were interviewed. The racial composition of the women's prison was approximately 82 percent white; therefore, the sample is considered representative of that population.[3] The men who responded to our survey were 64 percent white, which is identical to the proportion of overall prisoners; those who participated in interviews were 52.5 percent white, 17.5 percent Black, 20 percent Native American, 5 percent Hispanic, and 5 percent Other. The survey response rate for the men was significantly lower than for the women (49 percent of men versus 70 percent of women) and women of color were slightly underrepresented. The underrepresentation of Black, Indigenous, and other people of color is consistent with research that indicates that these groups tend to respond less frequently to survey research, given low levels of trust in the government and other official institutions.[4] Previous research also indicates that prescription drug use may be more common among white women, hence our slightly higher proportion of white women respondents.[5] Given that we asked for a random list of prisoners for the survey and responses were voluntary, we were unable to push for greater responses from women of color.

Some other limitations of our sample are due to sampling error. The men's sample skews older than a random sample because of a sampling error caused by prison officials when we asked for a random sample. The list oversampled lower prison inmate numbers, which reflects those who had been in the Department of Corrections for a longer period of time, thereby creating a sample of older offenders with longer offending histories. Our requirement that prisoners be incarcerated for less than five years meant these were men who had been in and out of prison. Unfortunately, we were unaware of this issue until the data had been collected. However, given the highest morbidity risk to older individuals, this sample may be even more adept at addressing our research questions.

Another important note is the high proportion of Native American men included in both our survey and interview samples. While Missouri correctional

TABLE A.1. Interview Demographics

Women Interview Sample (n = 40)			Men Interview Sample (n = 40)		
Age			Age		
18–25	4	10.0%	18–25	0	0.0%
26–35	20	50.0%	26–35	0	0.0%
36–45	13	32.5%	36–45	12	30.0%
46–55	3	7.5%	46–55	17	42.5%
56+	0	0.0%	56+	11	27.5%
Race			Race		
White	37	92.5%	White	21	52.5%
Black/African American	3	7.5%	Black/African American	7	17.5%
			Hispanic	2	5.0%
			Native American	8	20.0%
			Muslim	2	5.0%
Education			Education		
Less than high school	14	35.0%	Less than high school	7	17.5%
High school/GED	13	32.5%	High school/GED	26	65.0%
Some college	10	25.0%	Some college	6	15.0%
BA or higher	3	7.5%	BA or higher	1	2.5%

centers do not offer Native American as a racial category for prisoners in population reports, 8 percent of our survey respondents identified as Native American or American Indian, as did 20 percent of the men we interviewed, who were chosen based upon high incidence of prescription drug use. This disproportionately high number of Native American men in our interview pool reflects national trends of substance use as well as higher incarceration rates. Native Americans are incarcerated at a rate 38 percent higher than the general population. Further, substance use among Native Americans is much higher than among any other racial or ethnic group recorded by the Census. According to the 2013 National Survey on Drug Use and Health, 12.3 percent of American Indians were currently using illicit drugs, compared with 9.5 percent of whites, 8.8 percent of Hispanics, and 10.5 percent of African Americans.[6] Such high rates of substance use and incarceration reflect the historical legacies of poverty produced by US government displacement, disruption, and destruction of food systems and family networks and stability, and inadequate health care and education to compensate. As a result, Native Americans are much more likely to experience poverty and unemployment and tend to be underserved

Name	Age	Race	Education	Approx. # Arrests	# Children
Aiden	53	White	High school	>100	4
Braydon	42	White	Some college	>20	4
Cole	51	Black	Less than high school	40	14
Deante	47	Black	GED	30	5
Evan	41	White	GED	30	0
Frank	51	White, Native American	Some college	50	2
Gerardo	59	White	High school	120	0
Harry	42	White	GED	5	2
Isaac	48	White	GED	30–40	1
James	51	White	GED	>200	2
Kevin	47	White	GED	>100	5
Lonny	49	White, Native American	GED	20	>1
Michael	47	White	GED	13	4
Nick	45	Hispanic, Indian	High school	20	2
Oscar	37	White	Less than high school	30	3
Patrick	57	White, Native American	GED	700	1
Quentin	58	White	Less than high school	30	3
Raphael	42	White	GED	40–50	1
Steve	41	White	GED	25–30	4
Alejandro	53	White, Native American	GED	100	4
Bill	41	Native American	GED	20	0
Craig	42	Black	GED	15	1
Derrick	64	Black, Native American	Less than high school	4	4
Elvis	57	White	College degree	>50	4
Fareed	45	White	GED	Hundreds	2
Grant	53	White	GED	100	1
Henry	58	White	GED	8	1
Ivan	51	Hispanic	GED	10–15	1
Jerome	58	Black	GED	100	2
Kai	43	White	GED	30	1
Liam	60	Native American	Less than high school	60–70	10
Malachi	54	Black	Some college	20–30	4
Nehemiah	48	Black	GED	12–13	4

continued

Name	Age	Race	Education	Approx. # Arrests	# Children
Oliver	53	White	Some college	30	1
Paul	55	Black, Native American, White	GED	>50	16
Ronald	56	White	High school	12	1
Shaun	43	Black	Some college	15	9
Terrance	55	Black	Less than high school	250	0
Victor	63	White	Less than high school	100	3
Walter	65	Black	Some college	100	7

Note: All names of participants and identifying information have been altered to protect the privacy and confidentiality of their responses.

TABLE A.3. Women Interview Participants

Name	Age	Race	Education	Approx. # Arrests	# Children	Single Mother
Aliyah	31	Black	Graduate degree	5	1	Yes
Betsy	33	White	Less than high school	8	3	No
Carlotta	31	White	Some college	>5	3	No
Dee-Ann	39	White	Some college	2	2	Yes
Elizabeth	36	White	Some college	20	3	Yes
Fern	39	White	Less than high school	20	2	No
Gina	44	Black	Graduate degree	1	2	Yes
Helen	30	White	High school	5-7	3	Yes
Ingrid	39	White	High school	2	3	No
Jaclyn	30	White	Less than high school	40-50	1	Yes
Katie	27	White	High school	30	1	Yes
Lauren	30	White	Some college	20	5	No
Melissa	39	White	High school	30	3	No
Nancy	33	White	High school	15	2	Yes
Olivia	26	White	Less than high school	5	0	No
Pauline	32	White	High school	4	2	Yes
Rachel	27	White	Some college	6	3	Yes
Sara	22	White	Less than high school	10-15	0	No
Andrea	54	Black	Less than high school	14	1	No
Brittany	24	White	High school	4-5	0	No
Chelsea	37	White	Less than high school	20	2	Yes
Diana	33	White	Some college	>20	2	Yes
Eve	47	White	Less than high school	>13	3	No

Name	Age	Race	Education	Approx. # Arrests	# Children	Single Mother
Francis	39	White	Some college	1	3	No
Georgia	27	White	High school	30	1	Yes
Holly	27	White	High school	15	3	Yes
Irene	29	White	High school	>10	1	Yes
Janice	39	White	High school	20	3	No
Kelly	35	White	High school	>7	5	Yes
Lyndsey	45	White	Less than high school	6	2	Yes
Morgan	26	Black	Some college	12	1	No
Nicole	45	White	Some college	20	3	Yes
Olive	39	White	Less than high school	10	4	No
Penny	39	White	Less than high school	15	2	Yes
Rhianna	25	White	Less than high school	3-4	2	Yes
Stacey	32	White	Some college	>26	0	No
Tonya	49	White	High school	8	4	No
Veronica	27	White	Less than high school	13	0	No
Whitney	20	White	Less than high school	>10	0	No
Yolanda	34	White	College degree	>10	2	No

Note: All names of participants and identifying information have been altered to protect the privacy and confidentiality of their responses.

by the medical establishment, making them at a heightened risk for substance abuse. Accordingly, their overrepresentation in our sample reflects how they are disproportionately affected by the Rx drug epidemic or the prescription-to-prison pipeline.

Tables A.2 and A.3 provide more detailed demographic information for each of the interview respondents from each interview site: a men's or women's correctional facility. Each semistructured interview was recorded, transcribed verbatim, and analyzed in NVivo qualitative coding software in order to identify and categorize patterns that emerged in the narratives.[7] In using an iterative, grounded theory approach, I was able to identify and code patterns across narrative responses, identify logical contradictions that required greater analysis, and disentangle the various motivations and conceptualizations of different types of Rx use. This technique requires constant comparisons across codes and interviews in order to identify and code for emerging patterns.

We engaged in this iterative process of coding and analysis for the development of several academic papers. For this book, the data were delved into more deeply—tracing story lines within and across participants in order to understand how particular life events or intersecting factors such as gender, race, class, trauma, employment, or childbirth made some individuals more likely to use Rx drugs nonmedically or to suffer negative consequences. While these data are not intended (or able) to be used predictively or representatively or to identify causal links between such conditions and outcomes, they do offer insight into the lived perspectives of groups that have historically been marginalized and rendered invisible by all types of legislation as well as nationally funded research. This work is dedicated to these individuals who took the time to share their stories with us and who help us understand and offer solutions to the problems that they identified.

INTRODUCTION

1 News Network, "Nearly 7 in 10 Americans Take Prescription Drugs."
2 B. Smith, "Inappropriate Prescribing," 36; Han et al., "Prescription Opioid Use, Misuse."
3 Dumit, *Drugs for Life*.
4 Conrad and Schneider, *Deviance and Medicalization*.
5 Bronson and Carson, *Prisoners in 2017*.
6 Reuter, "Why Has US Drug Policy Changed So Little over 30 Years?"
7 Carson, *Prisoners in 2016*.
8 Hockenberry, Wachter, and Sladky, *Juvenile Residential Facility Census, 2014*.
9 Glaze and Maruschak, *Parents in Prison and Their Minor Children*.
10 Western and Pettit, *Collateral Costs*.
11 Substance Abuse and Mental Health Services Administration, *Key Substance Use and Mental Health Indicators in the United States* (2019), 1.
12 Substance Abuse and Mental Health Services Administration, *Key Substance Use and Mental Health Indicators in the United States* (2019), 18.
13 Drug Enforcement Administration, *Drugs of Abuse*.
14 The terms *abuse* and *misuse* are not used in this book given that they accomplish similar obfuscating effects as the terms *opioid epidemic* and *opioid crisis*. These terms obscure the ways in which nonmedical use can benefit rather than harm by characterizing behaviors in unequivocally negative terms. The terms *abuse* and *misuse* reflect a specific perspective—that of the medical and legal establishments who have the ability to police those boundaries. Pejorative terms such as *abuse* and *addict* impact the reader but also health-care practitioners and the individual using substances. For example, in a study of five hundred clinicians, researchers John Kelly and Cara Westerhoff found that clinicians who used such labels were more likely to treat their patients punitively than those who did not use these terms. As journalist Maia Szalavitz notes, the terms *substance abuse* and *substance abuser* imply that it is the individual using substances who is abusive and warranting punishment, not the environment that produced pain or harm in the first place.

See Kelly and Westerhoff, "Does It Matter How We Refer to Individuals with Substance-Related Conditions?"; Kelly, Dow, and Westerhoff, "Does Our Choice of Substance-Related Terms Influence Perceptions of Treatment Need?"; Szalavitz, *Unbroken Brain*.

15 Ranapurwala et al., "Opioid Overdose Mortality among Former North Carolina Inmates."

16 Garcia, *Pastoral Clinic*; McCorkel, *Breaking Women*; McKim, *Addicted to Rehab*.

17 In order to participate in a drug court, individuals must plead guilty to full charges—associated with harshest penalties. While they are spared these penalties if they follow the conditions of "treatment," if they fail—if they are caught with drugs in their system or violate their conditions of probation or parole—they are immediately sentenced to the fullest extent of the law. These sentences are often much more severe than if they had been able to enter into a plea bargain (or been able to successfully defend their innocence in the first place).

18 Garcia, *Pastoral Clinic*.

19 Brennan, Lohman, and Gwyther, "Access to Pain Management as a Human Right."

20 Norn, Kruse, and Kruse, "Opiumsvalmuen og morfin gennem tiderne."

21 N. Campbell, *OD*.

22 Watkins-Hayes, *Remaking a Life*.

23 N. Campbell, *OD*.

24 Kaye, *Enforcing Freedom*.

25 Berlant, "Slow Death (Sovereignty, Obesity, Lateral Agency)," 760.

26 Berlant, "Slow Death (Sovereignty, Obesity, Lateral Agency)," 764.

27 Berlant, "Slow Death (Sovereignty, Obesity, Lateral Agency)," 754.

28 Berlant, "Slow Death (Sovereignty, Obesity, Lateral Agency)," 760.

29 N. Campbell, *OD*.

30 Foucault, *History of Sexuality*.

31 Foucault, *Birth of Biopolitics*, 226, 228–30; Puar, *Right to Maim*, xviii, 13.

32 Zola, "Medicine as an Institution of Social Control"; Illich, *Medical Nemesis*.

33 Illich, *Medical Nemesis*, 7.

34 Casper and Morrison, "Medical Sociology and Technology."

35 Armstrong, "Rise of Surveillance Medicine."

36 Williams, Martin, and Gabe, "Pharmaceuticalisation of Society?"

37 Conrad, *Medicalization of Society*.

38 Abraham, "Pharmaceuticalization of Society in Context."

39 Loe, *Rise of Viagra*.

40 Abraham, "Pharmaceuticalization of Society in Context."

41 Ledley et al., "Profitability of Large Pharmaceutical Companies."

42 Rose, "Politics of Life Itself."

43 Puar, *Right to Maim*, xv.

44 Puar, *Right to Maim*, xv.

45 Wacquant, "Deadly Symbiosis."

46 Kaye, *Enforcing Freedom*, 22.

47 Wagner and Sawyer, "Whole Pie 2018."

48 Shelden, *Controlling the Dangerous Classes*, 143.

49 Pew Charitable Trusts, "More Imprisonment Does Not Reduce State Drug Problems."

50 M. Alexander, *New Jim Crow*, 186.

51 On this last point, see Benjamin, *Race after Technology*; O'Neil, *Weapons of Math Destruction*. On mandatory minimums and all-white juries, see M. Alexander, *New Jim Crow*, 109–16, 116–20. As an example of sentencing disparities, powder cocaine, commonly used among middle- and upper-class white populations, carries dramatically lighter sentencing guidelines than crack cocaine, which is cheaper and therefore more commonly used by working-class and poor Black populations. Despite it being the same substance, until the Fair Sentencing Act of 2010 passed by the Obama administration, the possession of five grams of crack cocaine was punished at the same severity as for five hundred grams of powder cocaine, resulting in a one-hundred-to-one disparity in legislation that conveniently mapped onto racial differences of substance use. While the Fair Sentencing Act reduced the disparity between the amount of crack cocaine in comparison to powder cocaine that triggers certain federal penalties, it remains at an eighteen-to-one weight ratio disparity. For more, see Provine, "Race and Inequality in the War on Drugs"; United States Sentencing Commission, *2015 Report to the Congress*.

52 M. Alexander, *New Jim Crow*, 199.

53 Larochelle et al., "Disparities in Opioid Overdose Death."

54 Conrad, "Medicalization and Social Control."

55 Chiarello, "Policing Pleasure"; Hatch, *Silent Cells*, 10–15, 91–93; Garcia, *Pastoral Clinic*; McCorkel, *Breaking Women*; McKim, *Addicted to Rehab*.

56 United States Department of Justice, *Drug Enforcement Administration (DEA) History 1980–1985*; Cole, *No Equal Justice*, 46–49.

57 Heitzeg, "Education or Incarceration."

58 United States Department of Education Office for Civil Rights, "2013–2014 Civil Rights Data Collection Data Snapshot."

59 Heitzeg, "Education or Incarceration"; Witt, "School Discipline Tougher on African Americans"; Wald and Losen, "Defining and Redirecting a School to Prison Pipeline"; Springer, "Interrupting the School-to-Prison Pipeline."

60 Neal and Rick, *Prison Boom*.

61 Harlow, *Education and Correctional Populations*; Stipek and Hanson, "Schools vs Prisons."

62 United States Department of Education, "State and Local Expenditures on Corrections and Education."

63 Mark, Levit, and Buck, "Datapoints"; Mojtabai and Olfson, "National Patterns in Antidepressant Treatment."

64 Rhee and Rosenheck, "Initiation of New Psychotropic Prescriptions."

65 Hatch, *Silent Cells*, 23.

66 Hatch, *Silent Cells*, 11–12; Abramsky and Fellner, *Ill-Equipped*; Gottschlich and Cetnar, "Drug Bills at Jail Top Food Costs."

67 Hashimoto, "Class Matters."

68 Schmitt, Reedt, and Blackwell, *Demographic Differences in Sentencing*.

69 Hatch, *Silent Cells*, 15–21.

70 Hatch, *Silent Cells*, 29–41.

71 Hatch, *Silent Cells*, 12.

72 Pager, *Marked*.

73 Hatch, *Silent Cells*, 16.

74 Equal Justice Initiative, "Racial Double Standard in Drug Laws."

75 Crenshaw, "Mapping the Margins"; P. Collins, *Black Feminist Thought*; Omi and Winant, *Racial Formation in the United States*.

76 P. Collins, *Black Feminist Thought*.

77 Crenshaw, "Mapping the Margins"; P. Collins, *Black Feminist Thought*; Omi and Winant, *Racial Formation in the United States*; Rothstein, *Color of Law*; Bonilla-Silva, *Racism without Racists*; Tatum, *Why Are All the Black Kids Sitting Together in the Cafeteria?*; Roberts, *Killing the Black Body*; Duster, "Race and Reification in Science"; Hatch, *Blood Sugar*; M. Alexander, *New Jim Crow*; Davis, *Are Prisons Obsolete?*

78 Coates, *Between the World and Me*.

79 The interviews are part of a broader study that was approved by the Institutional Review Board and received a certificate of confidentiality from the US National Institute on Drug Abuse that protects respondents' survey and interview responses. As of 2018, Missouri remained the only state without a prescription drug monitoring program, which may account for the particularly high rates of both medical and nonmedical Rx drug use.

80 Dumit, *Drugs for Life*; Conrad, *Medicalization of Society*; Conrad and Schneider, *Deviance and Medicalization*; Conrad, "Medicalization and Social Control"; Goffman, *Asylums*; Foucault, *Birth of the Clinic*; McCorkel, *Breaking Women*; Kaye, *Enforcing Freedom*; N. Campbell, *OD*; M. Alexander, *New Jim Crow*; McKim, *Addicted to Rehab*; Davis, *Are Prisons Obsolete?*

81 Bonilla-Silva, *Racism without Racists*.

82 Davis, *Are Prisons Obsolete?*

83 Sentencing Project, "State-by-State Data."

84 McCarthy, "Family Member Incarcerated."

85 Sentencing Project, "State-by-State Data: State Rankings."

86 Express Scripts, "America's State of Mind Report."

87 Kaiser Family Foundation, "Mental Health Care Health Professional Shortage Areas."

88 Agarwal and Landon, "Patterns in Outpatient Benzodiazepine Prescribing in the United States."

89 Centers for Disease Control and Prevention, "U.S. State Opioid Dispensing Rates."

90 Pager, *Marked*.

1. THE MEDICALIZATION AND CRIMINALIZATION OF PAIN

1 Brennan, Lohman, and Gwyther, "Access to Pain Management as a Human Right."

2 C. Martin et al., *Prescription Drug Use in the United States, 2015–2016*.

3 Centers for Disease Control and Prevention, "QuickStats: Percentage of Adults ≥ 18 Years."

4 Krebs, Carey, and Weinberger, "Accuracy of the Pain Numeric Rating."

5 W. Clark et al., "Unidimensional Pain Rating Scales."

6 Several studies have correlated patient satisfaction survey ratings and prescription of opioids: Sinnenberg et al., "What Factors Affect Physicians' Decisions to Prescribe Opioids in Emergency Departments?"; Vila et al., "Efficacy and Safety of Pain Management"; Zgierska, Rabago, and Miller, "Impact of Patient Satisfaction Ratings on Physicians and Clinical Care."

7 Scher et al., "Moving beyond Pain as the Fifth Vital Sign."

8 Bell and Salmon, "Pain, Physical Dependence and Pseudoaddiction"; Armstrong, "Rise of Surveillance Medicine"; Chiarello, "Law, Morality, and Health Care Professionals," 128.

9 Gross, "Presumed Dangerous."

10 Mitchell Cohen et al., "Ethical Perspectives."

11 Wailoo, *Pain.*

12 Meier, *Pain Killer*; Keefe, *Empire of Pain.*

13 Woolf et al., *How Are Income and Wealth Linked.*

14 Woolf et al., *How Are Income and Wealth Linked.*

15 Maciosek et al., "Greater Use of Preventive Services."

16 Finkelstein et al., "Oregon Health Insurance Experiment"; Chua and Sommers, "Changes in Health and Medical Spending"; Van der Wees, Zaslavsky, and Ayanian, "Improvements in Health Status after Massachusetts Health Care Reform"; Sommers et al., "Changes in Self-Reported Insurance Coverage." Perception of well-being may directly impact health itself. People who describe their health as "poor" have mortality rates two to ten times as high as those who report being in the healthiest category. In other words, perceptions of and experiences of health engage in a feedback loop whereby one directly impacts the other. For more, see Miilunpalo et al., "Self-Rated Health Status as a Health Measure"; DeSalvo et al., "Mortality Prediction with a Single General Self-Rated Health Question."

17 Yearby, "Racial Disparities in Health Status and Access to Healthcare."

18 Ellen, Mijanovich, and Dillman, "Neighborhood Effects on Health."

19 Walker, Keane, and Burke, "Disparities and Access to Healthy Food in the United States"; Larson, Story, and Nelson, "Neighborhood Environments"; Mobley et al., "Environment, Obesity, and Cardiovascular Disease Risk in Low-Income Women"; B. Clark, "Hospital Flight from Minority Communities."

20 Whiteis, "Hospital and Community"; Sager and Socolar, "Closing Hospitals in New York."

21 Sager, "Urban Hospital Closings"; Yearby, "Racial Disparities in Health Status and Access to Healthcare."

22 B. Clark, "Hospital Flight from Minority Communities."

23 Thomas and James, *Role of Health Coverage for Communities of Color.*

24 Yearby, "Racial Disparities in Health Status and Access to Healthcare"; Van Ryn et al., "Physicians' Perceptions of Patients' Social and Behavioral Characteristics"; Van Ryn and Burke, "Effect of Patient Race and Socio-economic Status."

25 Green et al., "Unequal Burden of Pain."

26 Petersen et al., "Vital Signs."

27 Centers for Disease Control and Prevention, "Racial and Ethnic Disparities Continue in Pregnancy-Related Deaths."

28 Ray et al., "Disparities in Time Spent Seeking Medical Care in the United States"; Ezenwa and Fleming, "Racial Disparities in Pain Management in Primary Care"; C. Campbell and Edwards, "Ethnic Differences in Pain and Pain Management"; Hewes et al., "Prehospital Pain Management."

29 Hill, Artiga, and Haldar, "Key Facts on Health and Health Care by Race and Ethnicity."

30 T. Lewis et al., "Perceived Discrimination and Blood Pressure in Older African American and White Adults"; Barnes et al., "Perceived Discrimination and Mortality in a Population-Based Study of Older Adults."

31 National Academies of Sciences, Engineering, and Medicine, *Growing Gap in Life Expectancy by Income*.

32 National Academies of Sciences, Engineering, and Medicine, *Growing Gap in Life Expectancy by Income*.

33 Western and Rosenfeld, "Unions, Norms, and the Rise in US Wage Inequality."

34 Courtwright, *Dark Paradise*.

35 Paulose-Ram et al., "Trends in Psychotropic Medication Use among US Adults."

36 Santo, Rui, and Ashman, "Physician Office Visits at Which Benzodiazepines Were Prescribed."

37 Johnson et al., "'Doing the Right Thing.'"

38 Quinones, *Dreamland*.

39 Clarke et al., "Biomedicalization"; Loe, *Rise of Viagra*; Smirnova, "Will to Youth."

40 Keefe, *Empire of Pain*, 40.

41 Keefe, *Empire of Pain*, 58, 161–62, 211.

42 Hong Kong also allows DTC advertising, and Brazil allows the advertisement of prescription drugs only in scientific, medical, or health professional journals. See Utsumi, "Advertising Regulation for Medication in Brazil"; "Undesirable Medical Advertisements Ordinance."

43 Guttmann, "Pharmaceutical Industry Direct to Consumer Spending."

44 Mikulic, "Prescription Drug Expenditure in the United States."

45 Mikulic, "Prescription Drug Expenditure in the United States."

46 DeJong et al., "Pharmaceutical Industry–Sponsored Meals"; Yeh et al., "Association of Industry Payments to Physicians."

47 Hadland et al., "Subsequent Opioid Prescribing."

48 Keefe, *Empire of Pain*, 211.

49 Meier, *Pain Killer*, 99; Porter and Jick, "Addiction Rare in Patients Treated with Narcotics"; Purdue Pharma, *OxyContin Marketing Plan, 2002*. Crucial to this promotion campaign was an obscure-turned-notorious letter to the editor that effectively convinced prescribers that risk of addiction to OxyContin was "less than one percent." The Porter and Jick letter was written to the editor of the prestigious medical journal the *New England Journal of Medicine* in 1980. This letter, submitted by Doctor Hershel Jick and his assistant, Jane Porter, came to establish the basis of

justification for the prescription of opioids to both hospitalized and nonhospitalized patients on the grounds that "the development of addiction is rare in medical patients." The letter read:

> To the Editor: Recently, we examined our current files to determine the incidence of narcotic addiction in 39,946 hospitalized medical patients who were monitored consecutively. Although there were 11,882 patients who received at least one narcotic preparation, there were only four cases of reasonably well documented addiction in patients who had a history of addiction. The addiction was considered major in only one instance. The drugs implicated were meperidine in two patients, Percodan in one, and hydromorphone in one. We conclude that despite widespread use of narcotic drugs in hospitals, the development of addiction is rare in medical patients with no history of addiction.
> Jane Porter
> Hershel Jick, M.D.
> Boston Collaborative Drug
> Surveillance Program
> Boston University Medical Center, Waltham MA 02154

Although this particular letter was one of many summary letters that Dr. Jick would submit to medical journals over his career, it was responsible for sparking a revolution in pain medication practice. In time, this single paragraph—buried in the back pages of a prestigious medical journal—came to be known simply as "Porter and Jick." From then on, the phrase "Porter and Jick" was a reference to the two claims attributed to the letter: (1) that less than 1 percent of patients treated with narcotics became addicted, and (2) that those who became addicted already had a "history of addiction." The letter was cited among pain specialists and nurses at conventions, seminars, and continuing medical education workshops to promote the idea that opiate painkillers were generally nonaddictive. The "less than 1 percent" statistic derived from this letter to the editor was cited widely, but with a crucial element of this statistic omitted. The number was based upon a database of *hospitalized patients* during a time when opiates were administered only (1) in small doses, (2) to those suffering acute pain, (3) in a hospital, and (4) under a doctor's supervision. These patients were not suffering from chronic pain or taking home bottles of pain pills. But those details were not captured in the "Porter and Jick" reference.

50 Keefe, *Empire of Pain*, 234.

51 Keefe, *Empire of Pain*, 264.

52 Booth, *Opium: A History*.

53 The nation's first drug law was actually aimed at white people who frequented opium dens in San Francisco's Chinatown and was enacted out of fear of racial mixing or, more specifically, that white women might form relationships with Chinese men. For more, see Provine, *Unequal under the Law*.

54 Legislators insisted that opium smoking was rampant among Chinese immigrants, yet these accusations were also dubious. In China, it was common to smoke opium

for holidays or special occasions but not to extremes or on a regular basis. Further, so-called opium dens quickly became popular among middle-class white people, serving more of this group than Chinese immigrants themselves. For more, see Courtwright, *Dark Paradise*.

55 Courtwright, *Dark Paradise*, 110.

56 Musto, *American Disease*, 11.

57 Hale, "When Jim Crow Drank Coke."

58 Anon, "Negro Cocaine Fiends."

59 Szalavitz, *Unbroken Brain*.

60 Bonnie and Whitebread, *Marijuana Conviction*; Michael Cohen, "Jim Crow's Drug War," 56–57.

61 For more on the power of controlling images, see P. Collins, *Black Feminist Thought*.

62 Kolb and Du Mez, "Drug Addiction in the United States and the Factors Influencing It"; Terry, "Drug Addictions, a Public Health Problem"; L. Brown, "Enforcement of the Tennessee Anti-narcotics Law."

63 Courtwright, *Dark Paradise*, 48.

64 Courtwright, *Dark Paradise*, 43.

65 Kaye, "Rehabilitating the 'Drugs Lifestyle.'"

66 Kaye, *Enforcing Freedom*, 23.

67 O. Lewis, "Culture of Poverty"; Kaye, "Rehabilitating the 'Drugs Lifestyle.'"

68 P. Collins, *Black Feminist Thought*, 69; Roberts, *Killing the Black Body*, 10–14.

69 Baum, "Legalize It All."

70 M. Alexander, *New Jim Crow*, 98.

71 *Economist*, "What Is the Most Dangerous Drug?"

72 M. Alexander, *New Jim Crow*.

73 Drug Policy Alliance, "History of the Drug War."

74 Baum, "Legalize It All."

75 Baum, "Legalize It All."

76 McKim, *Addicted to Rehab*.

77 Rosenberger, *America's Drug War Debacle*, 26.

78 While explicit mention of other mind-altering substances in the Bible is slim, one oft-cited passage prohibits "deeds of the flesh" such as "immorality, impurity, sensuality, idolatry, sorcery (*pharmakeia*), enmities, strife, jealousy, outbursts of anger, disputes, dissensions, factions, and envy; drunkenness, carousing, and the like" (Galatians 5:19). The passage denotes that "those who practice such things will not inherit the kingdom of God" (Galatians 5:20). *Pharmakeia*, one of these prohibited activities, is treated as a synonym for illicit substances or "poisons" associated with sorcery or witchcraft. In other words, those who use substances deemed illicit are, by definition, those who are immoral and not chosen by God. This circular logic extends the power to define and police the "just right" paradigm of substance use from the priest to the judge, as well as the doctor.

The Greek term *pharmakon*, from which both *pharmakeia* and the term *pharmaceutical* are derived, refers to both poisons and remedies. In fact, the etymology of the word reveals how the utility or danger of a substance is both context dependent and socially constructed. The concept of *pharmakeia* offers considerable insight into the history of mind-altering substances in the United States by drawing attention to the process by which a substance can be defined as a licit remedy in some contexts or for some individuals and as an illicit toxin for others.

The power afforded to certain social institutions to define the meaning of a substance is only further bolstered by biblical passages. For example, another excerpt instructs Christians to "drink no longer water, but use a little wine for thy stomach's sake and thine often infirmities" (Timothy 5:23). In this context, when a mind-altering substance is prescribed by a doctor it is moral and encouraged, as "it is necessary to submit to the authorities [of one's society], not only because of possible punishment but also as a matter of conscience" (Romans 13:1–5). Hence this religious text confers moral authority to doctors, legislators, and judges to distinguish what is legal or illegal, a remedy or a poison, but also what is moral or immoral. This has effectively expanded the power of separate institutions into a single interrelated authority structure that can dictate what is moral, as well as healthy and legal.

79 National Institute on Drug Abuse, "Drug Misuse and Addiction."
80 Garcia, *Pastoral Clinic*, 23.
81 McCorkel, *Breaking Women*, 85.
82 McCorkel, *Breaking Women*, 12.
83 Gowan and Whetstone, "Making the Criminal Addict," 87.
84 Kaye, *Enforcing Freedom*, 11.
85 Kaye, *Enforcing Freedom*, 10.
86 Garcia, *Pastoral Clinic*, 24.
87 On (1), see Berlant, "Slow Death (Sovereignty, Obesity, Lateral Agency)"; Puar, *Right to Maim*. On (2), see McCorkel, *Breaking Women*; McKim, *Addicted to Rehab*; Kaye, *Enforcing Freedom*. On (3), see Hatch, *Silent Cells*; N. Campbell, *OD*; M. Alexander, *New Jim Crow*.

2. PRESCRIPTION

1 Centers for Disease Control and Prevention, *National Health Interview Survey*.
2 Hales, Martin, and Gu, *Prevalence of Prescription Pain Medication Use among Adults*.
3 United Nations Development Programme, "Human Development Index."
4 Centers for Medicare and Medicaid Services, "Eligibility"; United States Department of Health and Human Services, "Who Is Eligible for Medicare?"
5 R. Cohen, Ward, and Schiller, *Health Insurance Coverage*.
6 Scott, "16,932 People Have Lost Medicaid Coverage."
7 Sapolsky, *Why Zebras Don't Get Ulcers*.
8 Acosta and Toro, "Let's Ask the Homeless People Themselves."
9 Elliott, Powell, and Brenton, "Being a Good Mom."
10 Bartky, "Foucault, Femininity, and the Modernization of Patriarchal Power"; Blum and Stracuzzi, "Gender in the Prozac Nation"; Fox and Neiterman, "Embodied Motherhood"; McKim, "Getting Gut-Level."

11 J. Martin et al., *Births*.

12 Morris, *Cut It Out*.

13 This figure may be an underestimation in our study given that we did not ask about childbirth in our interviews. During interviews, we asked individuals if they had ever been prescribed prescription drugs and for what ailments. The fact that over a third of them brought up a cesarean section indicates that others may have also been prescribed Rx drugs for a delivery but potentially did not mention it during their interview. It also highlights just how common childbirth may be as a pathway to nonmedical prescription drug use.

14 Morris, *Cut It Out*, 24.

15 Morris, *Cut It Out*, 19.

16 Morris, *Cut It Out*, 23.

17 C. Collins, *Making Motherhood Work*.

18 Khan et al., "I Didn't Want to Be 'That Girl.'"

19 S. Smith et al., *National Intimate Partner and Sexual Violence Survey*; Centers for Disease Control and Prevention, "NISVS: An Overview of 2010 Findings"; Walters, Chen, and Breiding, *National Intimate Partner and Sexual Violence Survey*.

20 Lisak et al., "False Allegations of Sexual Assault."

21 Pascoe and Hollander, "Good Guys Don't Rape," 69.

22 Browne, Miller, and Maguin, "Physical and Sexual Victimization among Incarcerated Women."

23 Kerker et al., "Adverse Childhood Experiences and Mental Health."

24 Substance Abuse and Mental Health Services Administration, *Results from the 2014 National Survey on Drug Use and Health*; National Institute of Mental Health, *Use of Mental Health Services and Treatment among Children*.

25 Anda et al., "Adverse Childhood Experiences and Prescribed Psychotropic Medications in Adults."

26 Hughes et al., "Effect of Multiple Adverse Childhood Experiences on Health"; Tonmyr and Shields, "Childhood Sexual Abuse and Substance Abuse"; Verona, Murphy, and Javdani, "Gendered Pathways."

27 Harvard University, *State of the Nation's Housing 2019*.

28 National Low Income Housing Coalition, "Out of Reach Report"; Joint Center for Housing Studies of Harvard University, "America's Rental Housing 2020."

29 Quinones, *Dreamland*, 255.

30 Quinones, *Dreamland*, 98.

3. PIPELINE

1 Hoffman et al., "Racial Bias in Pain Assessment"; Tamayo-Sarver et al., "Racial and Ethnic Disparities in Emergency Department Analgesic Prescription"; Winchester et al., "Racial and Ethnic Differences in Urine Drug Screening on Labor and Delivery"; Gaither et al., "Racial Disparities in Discontinuation of Long-Term Opioid Therapy."

2 Hoffman et al., "Racial Bias in Pain Assessment"; Ezenwa and Fleming, "Racial Disparities in Pain Management in Primary Care"; C. Campbell and Edwards,

"Ethnic Differences in Pain and Pain Management"; Hewes et al., "Prehospital Pain Management"; Kon, Pretzlaff, and Marcin, "Association of Race and Ethnicity with Rates of Drug and Alcohol Testing among US Trauma Patients"; M. Alexander, *New Jim Crow*, 109–14; Yearby, "Racial Disparities in Health Status and Access to Healthcare"; Myrick, Nelson, and Nielson, "Race and Representation."

3 Pager, *Marked*, 5, 31.

4 Pager, *Marked*, 101.

5 Hasin et al., "DSM-5 Criteria for Substance Use Disorders."

6 Hasin et al., "DSM-5 Criteria for Substance Use Disorders."

7 American Psychiatric Association, *Diagnostic and Statistical Manual of Mental Disorders*, 4th ed.

8 Garriott and Raikhel, "Addiction in the Making"; Vrecko, "Birth of a Brain Disease," 61.

9 Stafford, "Regulating Off-Label Drug Use," 1427.

10 Bell and Salmon, "Pain, Physical Dependence and Pseudoaddiction."

11 Courtwright, *Dark Paradise*, 43.

12 United States Department of Health and Human Services, *Sex, Race, and Ethnic Diversity of U.S. Health Occupations (2010–2012)*.

13 Pager, *Marked*, 31. Eighteen out of forty men and fourteen out of forty women referred to themselves in this way.

14 Pager, *Marked*, 5.

15 Frank et al., "Discrimination Based on Criminal Record."

16 Hampton, *American Fix*.

17 Smirnova and Owens, "Medicalized Addiction, Self-Medication, or Non-medical Prescription Drug Use?"

18 Chiarello, "Law, Morality, and Health Care Professionals," 128.

19 Meekosha and Jakubowicz, "Disability, Political Activism, and Identity Making"; Meekosha and Dowse, "Enabling Citizenship."

4. PRISON

1 These preliminary details were ones asked early on in the interview, and Andrea seemed to understand these questions and was able to respond accordingly. However, some of the later questions and details became more troublesome.

2 Torrey et al., *No Room at the Inn*; Sinclair, *Going, Going, Gone*.

3 Lamb and Weinberger, "Shift of Psychiatric Inpatient Care"; Wagner and Sawyer, "Whole Pie 2018."

4 Torrey et al., *Treatment of Persons with Mental Illness*; Torrey et al., *More Mentally Ill Persons Are in Jails*.

5 Hatch et al., "Soldier, Elder, Prisoner, Ward."

6 Abramsky and Fellner, *Ill-Equipped*; Bowen, Rogers, and Shaw, "Medication Management and Practices in Prison," 4.

7 Hatch, *Silent Cells*; Hatch et al., "Soldier, Elder, Prisoner, Ward."

8 Kim, Becker-Cohen, and Serakos, *Processing and Treatment of Mentally Ill Persons*.

9   It is also of note that seven of the twenty women who were diagnosed with a mental health issue were diagnosed with bipolar disorder. Given that interviewees were not specifically asked whether they had been diagnosed with a mental health issue, these figures are likely an underestimation.

10 Manderscheid, Atay, and Male, *Highlights of Organized Mental Health Services*, 243–79.

11 Bachrach, *Deinstitutionalization*; P. Brown, *Transfer of Care*; Warren, "New Forms of Social Control."

12 United States Department of Justice, Office of Justice Programs, "Bureau of Justice Statistics."

13 Social Security, "SSI Federal Payment Amounts."

14 Prins, "Does Transinstitutionalization Explain," 717.

15 Richie, *Compelled to Crime*.

16 Dworsky, Napolitano, and Courtney, "Homelessness during the Transition from Foster Care to Adulthood."

17 Gypen et al., "Outcomes of Children Who Grew Up in Foster Care"; Courtney et al., *Midwest Evaluation of the Adult Functioning of Former Foster Youth*; Hook and Courtney, "Employment Outcomes of Former Foster Youth"; Maliszewski and Brown, "Familism, Substance Abuse, and Sexual Risk among Foster Care Alumni."

18 Lindquist and Santavirta, "Does Placing Children in Out-of-Home Care Increase Their Adult Criminality?"

19 Children's Bureau, *AFCARS Report #28*.

20 Gypen et al., "Outcomes of Children Who Grew Up in Foster Care."

21 Dumit, *Picturing Personhood*, 5–8.

22 Pescosolido et al., "'Disease Like Any Other?'"

23 Phelan, "Geneticization of Deviant Behavior and Consequences for Stigma," 316.

24 McKim, *Addicted to Rehab*.

25 Garriott, *Policing Methamphetamine*.

26 Thielking, "Missouri Is the Only State."

27 Carson, *Prisoners in 2016*; Sentencing Project, "Trends in US Corrections."

28 Pager, *Marked*, 16–17.

29 Pager, *Marked*, 17.

30 Carson, *Prisoners in 2016*; Sentencing Project, "Trends in US Corrections"; United States Sentencing Commission, *Mandatory Minimum Penalties*.

31 Foucault, *Discipline and Punish*, 200–228; Bentham's panopticon is a circular prison with a guard tower in the center of the circular yard, where each prisoner is held in a cell without cell doors facing the center, yet no one runs because they are being watched and policed by everyone else, including themselves. If prisoners try to resist, they fear that someone else will turn them in, despite the fact that the prisoners vastly outnumber the guard and only with their cooperation can the system still exist. As a result, prisoners are kept captive by the physical boundaries of the institution, but also by internalized surveillance.

32 Penal Reform International, "Global Prison Trends 2021."

33 Reedt et al., *Recidivism among Federal Drug Trafficking Offenders*.

CONCLUSIONS

1   Ledley et al., "Profitability of Large Pharmaceutical Companies."
2   Busfield, "'Pill for Every Ill.'"
3   Sentencing Project, "State-by-State Data."
4   While there are individuals who give birth who are not women, in this study, all the interviewees who gave birth identified as women.
5   Nelson, *Body and Soul*, 11.
6   Nelson, *Body and Soul*, 12.
7   Chiarello, "War on Drugs Comes to the Pharmacy Counter."
8   Chiarello, "Where Movements Matter."
9   DeRubeis, Siegle, and Hollon, "Cognitive Therapy versus Medication for Depression."
10 United States Food and Drug Administration, "FDA Drug Safety Communication."
11 Wakeman et al., "Comparative Effectiveness of Different Treatment Pathways for Opioid Use Disorder."
12 National Center for Health Statistics, "Wide-Ranging Online Data for Epidemiologic Research."
13 Watkins-Hayes, *Remaking a Life*, 15–19.
14 Pager, *Marked*, 31–32.
15 Lopez, "Trump Administration."
16 Pollack and Reuter, "Does Tougher Enforcement Make Drugs More Expensive?"; Eisen, Roeder, and Bowling, "What Caused the Crime Decline?"
17 Carson, *Prisoners in 2016*; Sentencing Project, "Trends in US Corrections."
18 Phelps, "Paradox of Probation."
19 M. Alexander, *New Jim Crow*, 94. See also Pager, *Marked*.
20 Richie, *Compelled to Crime*; Garcia, *Pastoral Clinic*; Haney, *Offending Women*; Hatch, *Silent Cells*; Kaye, *Enforcing Freedom*; McCorkel, *Breaking Women*; McKim, *Addicted to Rehab*; Sue, *Getting Wrecked*; Tiger, *Judging Addicts*.
21 Drug Policy Alliance, "Making Economic Sense"; Pearl, "Ending the War on Drugs."
22 Davis, *Are Prisons Obsolete?*; Wilson, *Golden Gulag*; Shigematsu, *Visions of Abolition*; Kaba, "Being MK."
23 Wang, *Carceral Capitalism*.
24 Watkins-Hayes, *Remaking a Life*, 13.
25 Centers for Disease Control and Prevention, "Multiple Cause of Death."
26 M. Alexander, *New Jim Crow*, 192–95.
27 Kaye, *Enforcing Freedom*, 11; Steyee, *Program Performance Report*.
28 Edwards, "Saving Children, Controlling Families."
29 Haney, *Offending Women*, 224.
30 B. Alexander, "Myth of Drug-Induced Addiction."
31 Liu et al., "Social Bonding Decreases the Rewarding Properties of Amphetamine."

APPENDIX

1   Prison Policy Initiative, "Prison Wage Policies."
2   We sent 260 surveys to the men's institution, but 26 of the men's surveys were returned because they were undeliverable (e.g., the intended recipient had moved to another institution or had been released).
3   We were unable to find data on race by gender in the annual reports published by the Missouri Department of Corrections. We contacted the prison where data collection took place to get a record of the population number and racial distribution. Although these numbers fluctuate on a daily basis, we were informed that there were 1,250 white, 245 Black, and 28 Other women under supervision during the time of our interviews.
4   Schnittker, "Social Distance in the Clinical Encounter."
5   Broman, Miller, and Jackson, "Race-Ethnicity and Prescription Drug Misuse."
6   Substance Abuse and Mental Health Services Administration, *Results from the 2013 National Survey on Drug Use and Health.*
7   Strauss and Corbin, *Basics of Qualitative Research.*

BIBLIOGRAPHY

Abraham, John. "Pharmaceuticalization of Society in Context: Theoretical, Empirical and Health Dimensions." *Sociology* 44, no. 4 (2010): 603–22.

Abramsky, Sasha, and Jamie Fellner. *Ill-Equipped: US Prisons and Offenders with Mental Illness.* New York: Human Rights Watch, 2003.

Acosta, Olga, and Paul A. Toro. "Let's Ask the Homeless People Themselves: A Needs Assessment Based on a Probability Sample of Adults." *American Journal of Community Psychology* 28, no. 3 (2000): 343–66.

Agarwal, Sumit D., and Bruce E. Landon. "Patterns in Outpatient Benzodiazepine Prescribing in the United States." *JAMA Network Open* 2, no. 1 (2019): e187399. https://doi.org/10.1001/jamanetworkopen.2018.7399.

Alexander, Bruce K. "The Myth of Drug-Induced Addiction." Presentation to Senate of Canada, 2001. https://sencanada.ca/content/sen/committee/371/ille/presentation/alexander-e.htm.

Alexander, Michelle. *The New Jim Crow: Mass Incarceration in the Age of Colorblindness.* New York: New Press, 2010.

American Psychiatric Association. *Diagnostic and Statistical Manual of Mental Disorders.* 4th ed. Washington, DC: American Psychiatric Association, 1994.

Anda, Robert F., David W. Brown, Vincent J. Felitti, J. Douglas Bremner, Shanta R. Dube, and Wayne H. Giles. "Adverse Childhood Experiences and Prescribed Psychotropic Medications in Adults." *American Journal of Preventive Medicine* 32, no. 5 (2007): 389–94.

Anon. "Negro Cocaine Fiends." 1902. In *Drugs, Alcohol and Addiction in the Long Nineteenth Century*, vol. 2, *Healers Discovering and Treating Addiction*, edited by Dan Malleck, 152–53. London: Routledge, 2020.

Armstrong, David. "The Rise of Surveillance Medicine." *Sociology of Health and Illness* 17, no. 3 (1995): 393–404.

Bachrach, Leona L. *Deinstitutionalization: An Analytical Review and Sociological Perspective.* National Institute of Mental Health. Washington, DC: United States Government Printing Office, 1976.

Barnes, Lisa L., Carlos F. Mendes de Leon, Tené T. Lewis, Julia L. Bienias, Robert S. Wilson, and Denis A. Evans. "Perceived Discrimination and Mortality in a Population-Based Study of Older Adults." *American Journal of Public Health* 98, no. 7 (2008): 1241–47.

Bartky, Sandra L. "Foucault, Femininity, and the Modernization of Patriarchal Power." In *The Politics of Women's Bodies: Sexuality, Appearance, and Behavior*, edited by R. Weitz, 25–45. New York: Oxford University Press, 2003.

Baum, Dan. "Legalize It All: How to Win the War on Drugs." *Harper's Magazine*, April 2016, 21–32. https://harpers.org/archive/2016/04/legalize-it-all/.

Bell, Kirsten, and Amy Salmon. "Pain, Physical Dependence and Pseudoaddiction: Redefining Addiction for 'Nice' People?" *International Journal of Drug Policy* 20, no. 2 (2009): 170–78.

Benjamin, Ruha. *Race after Technology: Abolitionist Tools for the New Jim Code*. Harlow, UK: Penguin Books, 2019.

Berlant, Lauren. "Slow Death (Sovereignty, Obesity, Lateral Agency)." *Critical Inquiry* 33, no. 4 (2007): 754–80.

Blum, Linda M., and Nena F. Stracuzzi. "Gender in the Prozac Nation: Popular Discourse and Productive Femininity." *Gender and Society* 18, no. 3 (2004): 269–86.

Bonilla-Silva, Eduardo. *Racism without Racists: Color-Blind Racism and the Persistence of Racial Inequality in the United States*. 4th ed. Lanham, MD: Rowman and Littlefield, 2006.

Bonnie, Richard J., and Charles H. Whitebread II. *The Marijuana Conviction: A History of Marijuana Prohibition in the United States*. Charlottesville: University Press of Virginia, 1974.

Booth, Martin. *Opium: A History*. New York: St. Martin's, 1996.

Bowen, Robert A., Anne Rogers, and Jennifer Shaw. "Medication Management and Practices in Prison for People with Mental Health Problems: A Qualitative Study." *International Journal of Mental Health Systems* 3, no. 1 (2009): 1–11. https://doi.org/proxy .library.umkc.edu/10.1186/1752-4458-3-24.

Brennan, Frank, Diederik Lohman, and Liz Gwyther. "Access to Pain Management as a Human Right." *American Journal of Public Health* 109, no. 1 (2019): 61–65. https://doi.org /10.2105/AJPH.2018.304743.

Broman, Clifford L., Paula K. Miller, and Emmanuel Jackson. "Race-Ethnicity and Prescription Drug Misuse: Does Self-Esteem Matter?" *Journal of Child and Adolescent Behavior* 3, no. 5 (2015): 1–6.

Bronson, Jennifer, and E. Ann Carson. *Prisoners in 2017*. Washington, DC: Bureau of Justice Statistics, 2019.

Brown, Lucius P. "Enforcement of the Tennessee Anti-narcotics Law." *American Journal of Public Health* 5, no. 4 (1915): 323–33.

Brown, Phil, ed. *The Transfer of Care: Psychiatric Deinstitutionalization and Its Aftermath*. New York: Routledge, 1985.

Browne, Angela, Brenda Miller, and Eugene Maguin. "Prevalence and Severity of Lifetime Physical and Sexual Victimization among Incarcerated Women." *International Journal of Law and Psychiatry* 22, no. 3 (1999): 301–22.

Busfield, Joan. "'A Pill for Every Ill': Explaining the Expansion in Medicine Use." *Social Science and Medicine* 70, no. 6 (2010): 934–41.

Campbell, Claudia M., and Robert R. Edwards. "Ethnic Differences in Pain and Pain Management." *Pain Management* 2, no. 3 (2012): 219–30.

Campbell, Nancy D. *OD: Naloxone and the Politics of Overdose.* Cambridge, MA: MIT Press, 2020.

Carson, E. Ann. *Prisoners in 2016.* Washington, DC: Bureau of Justice Statistics, 2012.

Casper, Monica J., and Daniel R. Morrison. "Medical Sociology and Technology: Critical Engagements." Supplement, *Journal of Health and Social Behavior* 51, no. S1 (2010): S120–32.

Centers for Disease Control and Prevention. *Early Release of Selected Estimates Based on Data from the National Health Interview Survey.* National Center for Health Statistics, 2015. https://www.cdc.gov/nchs/data/nhis/earlyrelease/earlyrelease201605_11.pdf.

Centers for Disease Control and Prevention. "Multiple Cause of Death, 1999–2020." Request on CDC Wonder Online Database, 2020. Accessed January 21, 2021. http://wonder.cdc.gov/mcd-icd10.html.

Centers for Disease Control and Prevention. "NISVS: An Overview of 2010 Findings on Victimization by Sexual Orientation." National Center for Injury Prevention and Control, Division of Violence Prevention, 2011. Accessed August 28, 2018. https://www.cdc.gov/violenceprevention/pdf/cdc_nisvs_victimization_final-a.pdf.

Centers for Disease Control and Prevention. "Quickstats: Percentage of Adults ≥ 18 Years Who Often Had Pain in the Past 3 Months, *by Sex and Age Group—National Health Interview Survey, United States, 2010–2011." 2017. https://www.cdc.gov/mmwr/preview/mmwrhtml/mm6217a10.htm.

Centers for Disease Control and Prevention. "Racial and Ethnic Disparities Continue in Pregnancy-Related Deaths." September 5, 2019. https://www.cdc.gov/media/releases/2019/p0905-racial-ethnic-disparities-pregnancy-deaths.html.

Centers for Disease Control and Prevention. "U.S. State Opioid Dispensing Rates." 2012. https://www.cdc.gov/drugoverdose/rxrate-maps/state2012.html.

Centers for Medicare and Medicaid Services. "Eligibility." Medicaid.gov, 2022. Accessed February 11, 2022. https://www.medicaid.gov/medicaid/eligibility/index.html.

Chiarello, Elizabeth. "Law, Morality, and Health Care Professionals: A Multilevel Framework." *Annual Review of Law and Social Science* 15 (2019): 117–35.

Chiarello, Elizabeth. "Policing Pleasure: A Sociolegal Framework for Understanding the Social Control of Desire." In *Studies in Law, Politics, and Society,* vol. 73, edited by Austin Sarat, 109–39. Bingley, UK: Emerald, 2017.

Chiarello, Elizabeth. "The War on Drugs Comes to the Pharmacy Counter: Frontline Work in the Shadow of Discrepant Institutional Logics." *Law and Social Inquiry* 40, no. 1 (2015): 86–122.

Chiarello, Elizabeth. "Where Movements Matter: Examining Unintended Consequences of the Pain Management Movement in Medical, Criminal Justice, and Public Health Fields." *Law and Policy* 40, no. 1 (2018): 79–109.

Children's Bureau. *AFCARS Report #28.* November 19, 2021. https://www.acf.hhs.gov/cb/report/afcars-report-28.

Chua, Kao-Ping, and Benjamin D. Sommers. "Changes in Health and Medical Spending among Young Adults under Health Reform." *Journal of the American Medical Association* 311, no. 23 (2014): 2437–39.

Clark, Brietta R. "Hospital Flight from Minority Communities: How Our Existing Civil Rights Framework Fosters Racial Inequality in Healthcare." *DePaul Journal of Health Care Law* 9, no. 2 (2005): 1023–99.

Clark, W. Crawford, Joseph C. Yang, Siu-Lun Tsui, Kwok-Fu Ng, and Susanne Bennett Clark. "Unidimensional Pain Rating Scales: A Multidimensional Affect and Pain Survey (Maps) Analysis of What They Really Measure." *Pain* 98, no. 3 (2002): 241–47.

Clarke, Adele E., Janet K. Shim, Laura Mamo, Jennifer Ruth Fosket, and Jennifer R. Fishman. "Biomedicalization: Technoscientific Transformations of Health, Illness, and U.S. Biomedicine." *American Sociological Review* 68, no. 2 (2003): 161–94.

Coates, Ta-Nehisi. *Between the World and Me.* New York: Spiegel and Grau, 2015.

Cohen, Michael M. "Jim Crow's Drug War: Race, Coca Cola, and the Southern Origins of Drug Prohibition." *Southern Cultures* 12, no. 3 (2006): 55–79.

Cohen, Mitchell J. M., Samar Jasser, Patrick D. Herron, and Clorinda G. Margolis. "Ethical Perspectives: Opioid Treatment of Chronic Pain in the Context of Addiction." *Clinical Journal of Pain* 18, no. 4 (2002): S99–107.

Cohen, Robin A., Brian W. Ward, and Jeannine S. Schiller. *Health Insurance Coverage: Early Release of Estimates from the National Health Interview Survey, 2010.* Centers for Disease Control and Prevention, Division of Health Interview Statistics National Center for Health Statistics, 2011. Accessed August 28, 2018. https://www.cdc.gov/nchs/data/nhis/earlyrelease/insur201106.htm.

Cole, David. *No Equal Justice: Race and Class in the American Criminal Justice System.* New York: New Press, 1999.

Collins, Caitlin. *Making Motherhood Work: How Women Manage Careers and Caregiving.* Princeton, NJ: Princeton University Press, 2019.

Collins, Patricia Hill. *Black Feminist Thought: Knowledge, Consciousness, and the Politics of Empowerment.* New York: Routledge, 2000.

Conrad, Peter. "Medicalization and Social Control." *Annual Review of Sociology* 18, no. 1 (1992): 209–32.

Conrad, Peter. *The Medicalization of Society: On the Transformation of Human Conditions into Treatable Disorders.* Baltimore, MD: Johns Hopkins University Press, 2007.

Conrad, Peter, and Joseph W. Schneider. *Deviance and Medicalization: From Badness to Sickness.* St. Louis: Mosby, 1980.

Courtney, Mark E., Amy Lynn Dworsky, Gretchen Ruth Cusick, Judy Havlicek, Alfred Perez, and Thomas E. Keller. *Midwest Evaluation of the Adult Functioning of Former Foster Youth: Outcomes at Age 21.* Chicago: Chapin Hall Center for Children at the University of Chicago, 2007.

Courtwright, David T. *Dark Paradise: Opiate Addiction in America before 1940.* Cambridge, MA: Harvard University Press, 1982.

Crenshaw, Kimberlé. "Mapping the Margins: Intersectionality, Identity Politics, and Violence against Women of Color." *Stanford Law Review* 43, no. 6 (1991): 1241–99. https://doi.org/10.2307/1229039.

Davis, Angela. *Are Prisons Obsolete?* New York: Seven Stories, 2003.

DeJong, Colette, Thomas Aguilar, Chien-Wen Tseng, Grace A. Lin, W. John Boscardin, and R. Adams Dudley. "Pharmaceutical Industry–Sponsored Meals and Physician

Prescribing Patterns for Medicare Beneficiaries." *JAMA Internal Medicine* 176, no. 8 (2016): 1114–22.

DeRubeis, Robert J., Greg J. Siegle, and Steven D. Hollon. "Cognitive Therapy versus Medication for Depression: Treatment Outcomes and Neural Mechanisms." *Nature Reviews Neuroscience* 9, no. 10 (2008): 788–96.

DeSalvo, Karen B., Nicole Bloser, Kristi Reynolds, Jiang He, and Paul Muntner. "Mortality Prediction with a Single General Self-Rated Health Question." *Journal of General Internal Medicine* 21, no. 3 (2006): 267–75.

Drug Enforcement Administration. *Drugs of Abuse: A DEA Resource Guide; 2017 Edition.* United States Department of Justice, Drug Enforcement Administration, 2017. https://www.dea.gov/sites/default/files/drug_of_abuse.pdf.

Drug Policy Alliance. "A History of the Drug War." 2022. Accessed January 21, 2021. https://drugpolicy.org/issues/brief-history-drug-war.

Drug Policy Alliance. "Making Economic Sense." Drug Policy Alliance, 2022. Accessed January 21, 2022. https://drugpolicy.org/issues/making-economic-sense.

Dumit, Joseph. *Drugs for Life: How Pharmaceutical Companies Define Our Health.* Durham, NC: Duke University Press, 2012.

Dumit, Joseph. *Picturing Personhood: Brain Scans and Biomedical Identity.* Princeton, NJ: Princeton University Press, 2004.

Duster, Troy. "Race and Reification in Science." *Science* 307, no. 512 (2005): 1050–51. https://doi.org/10.1126/science.1110303.

Dworsky, Amy, Laura Napolitano, and Mark Courtney. "Homelessness during the Transition from Foster Care to Adulthood." Supplement, *American Journal of Public Health* 103, no. S2 (2013): S318–23.

Economist. "What Is the Most Dangerous Drug?" June 25, 2019. https://www.economist.com/graphic-detail/2019/06/25/what-is-the-most-dangerous-drug.

Edwards, Frank. "Saving Children, Controlling Families: Punishment, Redistribution, and Child Protection." *American Sociological Review* 81, no. 3 (2016): 575–95.

Eisen, Lauren-Brooke, Olivia Roeder, and Julia Bowling. "What Caused the Crime Decline?" Brennan Center for Justice, February 15, 2015. https://www.brennancenter.org/publication/what-caused-crime-decline.

Ellen, Ingrid Gould, Tod Mijanovich, and Keri-Nicole Dillman. "Neighborhood Effects on Health: Exploring the Links and Assessing the Evidence." *Journal of Urban Affairs* 23, nos. 3–4 (2001): 391–408.

Elliott, Sinikka, Rachel Powell, and Joslyn Brenton. "Being a Good Mom: Low-Income, Black Single Mothers Negotiate Intensive Mothering." *Journal of Family Issues* 36, no. 3 (February 2015): 351–70. https://doi.org/10.1177/0192513X13490279.

Equal Justice Initiative. "Racial Double Standard in Drug Laws Persists Today." December 19, 2019. https://eji.org/news/racial-double-standard-in-drug-laws-persists-today/.

Express Scripts. "America's State of Mind Report." Evernorth Health Inc., April 16, 2020. https://www.express-scripts.com/corporate/americas-state-of-mind-report.

Ezenwa, Miriam, and M. Fleming. "Racial Disparities in Pain Management in Primary Care." *Journal of Pain* 5, no. 3 (2012): 12–26.

Finkelstein, Amy, Sarah Taubman, Bill Wright, Mira Bernstein, Jonathan Gruber, Joseph P. Newhouse, Heidi Allen, Katherine Baicker, and Oregon Health Study Group. "The Oregon Health Insurance Experiment: Evidence from the First Year." *Quarterly Journal of Economics* 127, no. 3 (2012): 1057–106.

Foucault, Michel. *The Birth of Biopolitics: Lectures at the Collège de France, 1978–1979*. Edited by Michel Senellart. Translated by Graham Burchell. Basingstoke, UK: Palgrave Macmillan, 2008.

Foucault, Michel. *The Birth of the Clinic: An Archaeology of Medical Perception*. New York: Vintage Books, 1975.

Foucault, Michel. *Discipline and Punish: The Birth of the Prison*. New York: Vintage Books, 2012.

Foucault, Michel. *The History of Sexuality, Volume 1*. New York: Vintage, 1990.

Fox, Bonnie, and Elena Neiterman. "Embodied Motherhood: Women's Feelings about Their Postpartum Bodies." *Gender and Society* 29, no. 9 (2015): 670–93.

Frank, Joseph W., Emily A. Wang, Marcella Nunez-Smith, Hedwig Lee, and Megan Comfort. "Discrimination Based on Criminal Record and Healthcare Utilization among Men Recently Released from Prison: A Descriptive Study." *Health and Justice* 2, no. 1 (2014): 1–8.

Gaither, Julie R., Kirsha Gordon, Stephen Crystal, E. Jennifer Edelman, Robert D. Kerns, Amy C. Justice, David A. Fiellin, and William C. Becker. "Racial Disparities in Discontinuation of Long-Term Opioid Therapy following Illicit Drug Use among Black and White Patients." *Drug and Alcohol Dependence* 192 (November 2018): 371–76.

Garcia, Angela N. *The Pastoral Clinic: Addiction and Dispossession along the Rio Grande*. Berkeley: University of California Press, 2007.

Garriott, William. *Policing Methamphetamine: Narcopolitics in Rural America*. New York: New York University Press, 2011.

Garriott, William, and Eugene Raikhel. "Addiction in the Making." *Annual Review of Anthropology* 44 (2015): 477–91.

Glaze, Lauren E., and Laura M. Maruschak. *Parents in Prison and Their Minor Children: Survey of Prison Inmates*. Washington, DC: Bureau of Justice Statistics, 2016.

Goffman, Erving. *Asylums: Essays on the Social Situation of Mental Patients and Other Inmates*. Garden City, NY: Anchor Books, 1961.

Gottschlich, A. J., and G. Cetnar. "Drug Bills at Jail Top Food Costs." *Springfield [OH] News-Sun*, August 20, 2002.

Gowan, Teresa, and Sarah Whetstone. "Making the Criminal Addict: Subjectivity and Social Control in a Strong-Arm Rehab." *Punishment and Society* 14, no. 1 (2012): 69–93.

Green, Carmen R., Karen O. Anderson, Tamara A. Baker, Lisa C. Campbell, Sheila Decker, Roger B. Fillingim, Donna A. Kaloukalani, et al. "The Unequal Burden of Pain: Confronting Racial and Ethnic Disparities in Pain." *Pain Medicine* 4, no. 3 (2003): 277–94.

Gross, David E. "Presumed Dangerous: California's Selective Policy of Forcibly Medicating State Prisoners with Antipyschotic Drugs." *UC Davis Law Review* 35 (January 2001): 483–517.

Guttmann, A. "Pharmaceutical Industry Direct to Consumer Spending on Traditional Media in the United States from 2016 to 2020." Statista, May 11, 2021. https://www.statista.com/statistics/317819/pharmaceutical-industry-dtc-media-spending-usa/.

Gypen, Laura, Johan Vanderfaeillie, Skrallan De Maeyer, Laurence Belenger, and Frank Van Holen. "Outcomes of Children Who Grew Up in Foster Care: Systematic-Review." *Children and Youth Services Review* 76 (May 2017): 74–83.

Hadland, Scott E., Magdalena Cerdá, Yu Li, Maxwell S. Krieger, and Brandon D. L. Marshall. "Association of Pharmaceutical Industry Marketing of Opioid Products to Physicians with Subsequent Opioid Prescribing." *JAMA Internal Medicine* 178, no. 6 (2018): 861–63.

Hale, Grace Elizabeth. "When Jim Crow Drank Coke." *New York Times*, January 28, 2013. https://www.nytimes.com/2013/01/29/opinion/when-jim-crow-drank-coke.html.

Hales, Craig M., Crescent B. Martin, and Qiuping Gu. *Prevalence of Prescription Pain Medication Use among Adults: United States, 2015–2018.* United States Department of Health and Human Services, Centers for Disease Control and Prevention. Hyattsville, MD: National Center for Health Statistics, 2020.

Hampton, Ryan. *American Fix: Inside the Opioid Addiction Crisis—and How to End It.* New York: All Points Books, 2018.

Han, Beth, Wilson M. Compton, Carlos Blanco, Elizabeth Crane, Jinhee Lee, and Christopher M. Jones. "Prescription Opioid Use, Misuse, and Use Disorders in U.S. Adults: 2015 National Survey on Drug Use and Health." *Annals of Internal Medicine* 167, no. 5 (2017): 293–301.

Haney, Lynne. *Offending Women: Power, Punishment, and the Regulation of Desire.* Berkeley: University of California Press, 2010.

Harlow, Caroline Wolf. *Education and Correctional Populations.* Bureau of Justice Statistics Special Report. Washington, DC: United States Department of Justice Office of Justice Programs, 2003. https://www.bjs.gov/content/pub/pdf/ecp.pdf.

Harvard University. *The State of the Nation's Housing 2019.* Joint Center for Housing Studies of Harvard University, 2019. Accessed March 2, 2020. https://www.jchs.harvard.edu/state-nations-housing-2019.

Hashimoto, Erica J. "Class Matters." *Journal of Criminal Law and Criminology* 101, no. 1 (2013): 31.

Hasin, Deborah S., Charles P. O'Brien, Marc Auriacombe, Guilherme Borges, Kathleen Bucholz, Alan Budney, Wilson M. Compton, et al. "DSM-5 Criteria for Substance Use Disorders: Recommendations and Rationale." *American Journal of Psychiatry* 170, no. 8 (2013): 834–51.

Hatch, Anthony R., Marik Xavier-Brier, Brandon Attell, and Eryn Viscarra. "Soldier, Elder, Prisoner, Ward: Psychotropics in the Era of Transinstitutionalization." In *50 Years after Deinstitutionalization: Mental Illness in Contemporary Communities*, edited by Brea L. Perry, 291–317. Bingley, UK: Emerald, 2016.

Hatch, Anthony Ryan. *Blood Sugar: Racial Pharmacology and Food Injustice in America.* Minneapolis: University of Minnesota Press, 2016.

Hatch, Anthony Ryan. *Silent Cells: The Secret Drugging of Captive America.* Minneapolis: University of Minnesota Press, 2019.

Heitzeg, Nancy A. "Education or Incarceration: Zero Tolerance Policies and the School to Prison Pipeline." Paper presented at the Forum on Public Policy Online, 2009.

Hewes, Hilary A., Mengtao Dai, N. Clay Mann, Tanya Baca, and Peter Taillac. "Prehospital Pain Management: Disparity by Age and Race." *Prehospital Emergency Care* 22, no. 2 (2018): 189–97.

Hill, Latoya, Samantha Artiga, and Sweta Haldar. "Key Facts on Health and Health Care by Race and Ethnicity." Henry Kaiser Family Foundation, 2016. https://www.kff.org/report-section/key-facts-on-health-and-health-care-by-race-and-ethnicity-section-2-health-access-and-utilization/.

Hockenberry, Sarah, Andrew Wachter, and Anthony Sladky. *Juvenile Residential Facility Census, 2014*. US Department of Justice, Office of Juvenile Justice and Delinquency Prevention (OJJDP). National Report Series Bulletin: 2016. https://www.ojjdp.gov/pubs/250123.pdf.

Hoffman, Kelly M., Sophie Trawalter, Jordan R. Axt, and M. Norman Oliver. "Racial Bias in Pain Assessment and Treatment Recommendations, and False Beliefs about Biological Differences between Blacks and Whites." *Proceedings of the National Academy of Sciences* 113, no. 16 (2016): 4296–301.

Hook, Jennifer L., and Mark E. Courtney. "Employment Outcomes of Former Foster Youth as Young Adults: The Importance of Human, Personal, and Social Capital." *Children and Youth Services Review* 33, no. 10 (2011): 1855–65.

Hughes, Karen, Mark A. Bellis, Katherine A. Hardcastle, Dinesh Sethi, Alexander Butchart, Christopher Mikton, Lisa Jones, and Michael P. Dunne. "The Effect of Multiple Adverse Childhood Experiences on Health: A Systematic Review and Meta-analysis." *Lancet Public Health* 2, no. 8 (2017): e356–66.

Human Reproduction Programme. "WHO Statement of Cesarean Section Rates." Geneva: World Health Organization, 2015. https://apps.who.int/iris/bitstream/handle/10665/161442/WHO_RHR_15.02_eng.pdf?sequence=1.

Illich, Ivan. *Medical Nemesis: The Expropriation of Health*. London: Calder and Boyars, 1975.

Johnson, Chris F., Brian Williams, Stephen A. MacGillivray, Nadine J. Dougall, and Margaret Maxwell. "'Doing the Right Thing': Factors Influencing GP Prescribing of Antidepressants and Prescribed Doses." *BMC Family Practice* 18, no. 1 (2017): 1–13.

Joint Center for Housing Studies of Harvard University. "America's Rental Housing 2020." 2020. https://www.jchs.harvard.edu/sites/default/files/reports/files/Harvard_JCHS_Americas_Rental_Housing_2020.pdf.

Kaba, Mariame. "Being MK: My Personal Website." Accessed May 20, 2021. http://mariamekaba.com/.

Kaiser Family Foundation. "Mental Health Care Health Professional Shortage Areas." Henry Kaiser Family Foundation, 2021. https://www.kff.org/other/state-indicator/mental-health-care-health-professional-shortage-areas-hpsas/.

Kaye, Kerwin. *Enforcing Freedom: Drug Courts, Therapeutic Communities, and the Intimacies of the State*. New York: Columbia University Press, 2019.

Kaye, Kerwin. "Rehabilitating the 'Drugs Lifestyle': Criminal Justice, Social Control, and the Cultivation of Agency." *Ethnography* 14, no. 2 (2013): 207–32.

Keefe, Patrick Radden. *Empire of Pain*. New York: Doubleday, 2021.

Kelly, John F., and Cassandra M. Westerhoff. "Does It Matter How We Refer to Individuals with Substance-Related Conditions? A Randomized Study of Two Commonly Used Terms." *International Journal of Drug Policy* 21, no. 3 (2010): 202–7.

Kelly, John F., Sarah J. Dow, and Cara Westerhoff. "Does Our Choice of Substance-Related Terms Influence Perceptions of Treatment Need? An Empirical Investigation with Two Commonly Used Terms." *Journal of Drug Issues* 40, no. 4 (2010): 805–18.

Kerker, Bonnie D., Jinjin Zhang, Erum Nadeem, Ruth E. K. Stein, Michael S. Hurlburt, Amy Heneghan, John Landsverk, and Sarah McCue Horwitz. "Adverse Childhood Experiences and Mental Health, Chronic Medical Conditions, and Development in Young Children." *Academic Pediatrics* 15, no. 5 (2015): 510–17.

Khan, Shamus R., Jennifer S. Hirsch, Alexander Wambold, and Claude A. Mellins. "'I Didn't Want to Be "That Girl"': The Social Risks of Labeling, Telling, and Reporting Sexual Assault." *Sociological Science* 5 (July 2018): 432–60.

Kim, KiDeuk, Miriam Becker-Cohen, and Maria Serakos. *The Processing and Treatment of Mentally Ill Persons in the Criminal Justice System: A Scan of Practice and Background Analysis.* Washington, DC: Urban Institute, 2015.

Kolb, Lawrence, and Andrew Grover Du Mez. "The Prevalence and Trend of Drug Addiction in the United States and the Factors Influencing It." *Public Health Reports (1896–1970)* 39, no. 21 (1924): 1179–204.

Kon, Alexander A., Robert K. Pretzlaff, and James P. Marcin. "The Association of Race and Ethnicity with Rates of Drug and Alcohol Testing among US Trauma Patients." *Health Policy* 69, no. 2 (2004): 159–67.

Krebs, Erin E., Timothy S. Carey, and Morris Weinberger. "Accuracy of the Pain Numeric Rating Scale as a Screening Test in Primary Care." *Journal of General Internal Medicine* 22, no. 10 (2007): 1453–58.

Lamb, H. Richard, and Linda E. Weinberger. "The Shift of Psychiatric Inpatient Care from Hospitals to Jails and Prisons." *Journal of the American Academy of Psychiatry and the Law Online* 33, no. 4 (2005): 529–34.

Larochelle, Marc R., Svetla Slavova, Elisabeth D. Root, Daniel J. Feaster, Patrick J. Ward, Sabrina C. Selk, Charles Knott, Jennifer Villani, and Jeffrey H. Samet. "Disparities in Opioid Overdose Death Trends by Race/Ethnicity, 2018–2019, from the HEALing Communities Study." *American Journal of Public Health* 111, no. 10 (2021): 1851–54.

Larson, Nicole I., Mary T. Story, and Melissa C. Nelson. "Neighborhood Environments: Disparities in Access to Healthy Foods in the U.S." *American Journal of Preventive Medicine* 36, no. 1 (2009): 74–81.

Ledley, F. D., S. S. McCoy, G. Vaughan, and E. K. Cleary. "Profitability of Large Pharmaceutical Companies Compared with Other Large Public Companies." *Journal of the American Medical Association* 323, no. 9 (2020): 834–43.

Lewis, Oscar. "The Culture of Poverty." *Scientific American* 215, no. 4 (1966): 19–25.

Lewis, Tené T., Lisa L. Barnes, Julia L. Bienias, Daniel T. Lackland, Denis A. Evans, and Carlos F. Mendes de Leon. "Perceived Discrimination and Blood Pressure in Older African American and White Adults." *Journals of Gerontology Series A: Biomedical Sciences and Medical Sciences* 64, no. 9 (2009): 1002–8.

Lindquist, Matthew J., and Torsten Santavirta. "Does Placing Children in Out-of-Home Care Increase Their Adult Criminality?" *Labour Economics* 31 (October 2014): 72–83.

Lisak, David, Lori Gardinier, Sarah C. Nicksa, and Ashley M. Cote. "False Allegations of Sexual Assault: An Analysis of Ten Years of Reported Cases." *Violence against Women* 16, no. 12 (2010): 1318–34.

Liu, Yan, Kimberly A. Young, J. Thomas Curtis, Brandon J. Aragona, and Zuoxin Wang. "Social Bonding Decreases the Rewarding Properties of Amphetamine through a Dopamine D1 Receptor-Mediated Mechanism." *Journal of Neuroscience* 31, no. 22 (2011): 7960–66.

Loe, Meika. *The Rise of Viagra: How the Little Blue Pill Changed Sex in America*. New York: New York University Press, 2004.

Lopez, German. "The Trump Administration Just Took Its First Big Step to Escalate the War on Drugs." *Vox*, May 12, 2017. https://www.vox.com/policy-and-politics/2017/5/12/15597632/trump-sessions-war-on-drugs.

Maciosek, Michael V., Ashley B. Coffield, Thomas J. Flottemesch, Nichol M. Edwards, and Leif I. Solberg. "Greater Use of Preventive Services in US Health Care Could Save Lives at Little or No Cost." *Health Affairs* 29, no. 9 (2010): 1656–60.

Maliszewski, Genevieve, and Chris Brown. "Familism, Substance Abuse, and Sexual Risk among Foster Care Alumni." *Children and Youth Services Review* 36 (January 2014): 206–12.

Manderscheid, Ronald W., Joanne E. Atay, and A. Male. *Highlights of Organized Mental Health Services in 2000 and Major National and State Trends*. Washington, DC: Center for Mental Health Services, 2002.

Mark, Tami L., Katharine R. Levit, and Jeffrey A. Buck. "Datapoints: Psychotropic Drug Prescriptions by Medical Specialty." *Psychiatric Services* 60, no. 9 (2009): 1167. https://doi.org/10.1176/ps.2009.60.9.1167.

Martin, Crescent B., Craig M. Hales, Qiuping Gu, and Cynthia L. Ogden. *Prescription Drug Use in the United States, 2015–2016*. Hyattsville, MD: National Center for Health Statistics, 2019.

Martin, Joyce A., Brady E. Hamilton, Michelle J. K. Osterman, Sally C. Curtin, and T. J. Matthews. *Births: Final Data for 2013*. Centers for Disease Control and Prevention. Hyattsville, MD: National Center for Health Statistics, 2012.

McCarthy, Niall. "Over Half of Americans Have Had a Family Member Incarcerated." *Forbes*, December 7, 2018. https://www.forbes.com/sites/niallmccarthy/2018/12/07/over-half-of-americans-have-had-a-family-member-incarcerated-infographic/?sh=7184cf0f3e4f.

McCorkel, Jill A. *Breaking Women: Gender, Race, and the New Politics of Imprisonment*. New York: New York University Press, 2013.

McKim, Allison. *Addicted to Rehab: Race, Gender, and Drugs in the Era of Mass Incarceration*. New Brunswick, NJ: Rutgers University Press, 2017.

McKim, Allison. "Getting Gut-Level: Punishment, Gender, and Therapeutic Governance." *Gender and Society* 22, no. 3 (2008): 303–23.

Meekosha, Helen, and Leanne Dowse. "Enabling Citizenship: Gender, Disability and Citizenship in Australia." *Feminist Review* 57, no. 1 (Autumn 1997): 49–72.

Meekosha, Helen, and Andrew Jakubowicz. "Disability, Political Activism, and Identity Making: A Critical Feminist Perspective on the Rise of Disability Movements in Australia, the USA, and the UK." *Disability Studies Quarterly* 19, no. 4 (2000): 393–404.

Meier, Barry. *Pain Killer*. Emmaus, PA: Rodale, 2003.

Miilunpalo, Seppo, Ilkka Vuori, Pekka Oja, Matti Pasanen, and Helka Urponen. "Self-Rated Health Status as a Health Measure: The Predictive Value of Self-Reported Health Status on the Use of Physician Services and on Mortality in the Working-Age Population." *Journal of Clinical Epidemiology* 50, no. 5 (1997): 517–28.

Mikulic, Matej. "Prescription Drug Expenditure in the United States from 1960 to 2020." Statista, January 14, 2022. https://www.statista.com/statistics/184914/prescription -drug-expenditures-in-the-us-since-1960/.

Mobley, Lee R., Elisabeth D. Root, Eric A. Finkelstein, Olga Khavjou, Rosanne P. Farris, and Julie C. Will. "Environment, Obesity, and Cardiovascular Disease Risk in Low-Income Women." *American Journal of Preventive Medicine* 30, no. 4 (2006): 327–32.

Mojtabai, Ramin, and Mark Olfson. "National Patterns in Antidepressant Treatment by Psychiatrists and General Medical Providers: Results from the National Comorbidity Survey Replication." *Journal of Clinical Psychiatry* 69, no. 7 (2008): 1064–74.

Morris, Theresa. *Cut It Out: The C-Section Epidemic in America*. New York: New York University Press, 2016.

Musto, David F. *The American Disease: Origins of Narcotic Control*. New York: Oxford University Press, 1987.

Myrick, Amy, Robert L. Nelson, and Laura Beth Nielson. "Race and Representation: Racial Disparities in Legal Representation for Employment Civil Rights Plaintiffs." *New York University Journal of Legislation and Public Policy* 15, no. 3 (2012): 705–58.

National Academies of Sciences, Engineering, and Medicine. *The Growing Gap in Life Expectancy by Income: Implications for Federal Programs and Policy Responses*. Washington, DC: National Academies Press, 2015. https://nap.nationalacademies.org/read/19015 /chapter/1.

National Center for Health Statistics. "Wide-Ranging Online Data for Epidemiologic Research." Atlanta, GA: Centers for Disease Control and Prevention, 2020. https:// wonder.cdc.gov/wonder/help/main.html.

National Institute of Mental Health. *Use of Mental Health Services and Treatment among Children*. 2020. Accessed February 11, 2020. http://www.nimh.nih.gov/health/statistics /prevalence/use-of-mental-health-services-and-treatment-among-children.shtml.

National Institute on Drug Abuse. "Drug Misuse and Addiction." July 13, 2020. https:// nida.nih.gov/publications/drugs-brains-behavior-science-addiction/drug-misuse -addiction.

National Low Income Housing Coalition. "Out of Reach Report." 2019. https://reports .nlihc.org/sites/default/files/oor/OOR_2019.pdf.

Neal, Derek, and Armin Rick. *The Prison Boom and the Lack of Black Progress after Smith and Welch*. Cambridge, MA: National Bureau of Economic Research, 2014. http://www .nber.org/papers/w20283.

Nelson, Alondra. *Body and Soul: The Black Panther Party and the Fight against Medical Discrimination*. Minneapolis: University of Minnesota Press, 2013.

News Network. "Nearly 7 in 10 Americans Take Prescription Drugs, Mayo Clinic, Olmsted Medical Center Find." June 19, 2013. https://newsnetwork.mayoclinic.org/discussion/nearly-7-in-10-americans-take-prescription-drugs-mayo-clinic-olmsted-medical-center-find/.

Norn, S., P. R. Kruse, and E. Kruse. "Opiumsvalmuen og morfin gennem tiderne." *Dansk Medicinhistorisk Arborg* 33 (2005): 171–84.

Omi, Michael, and Howard Winant. *Racial Formation in the United States.* New York: Routledge, 2014.

O'Neil, Cathy. *Weapons of Math Destruction.* Harlow, UK: Penguin, 2017.

Pager, Devah. *Marked: Race, Crime, and Finding Work in an Era of Mass Incarceration.* Chicago: University of Chicago Press, 2008.

Pascoe, Cheri Jo, and Jocelyn A Hollander. "Good Guys Don't Rape: Gender, Domination, and Mobilizing Rape." *Gender and Society* 30, no. 1 (2016): 67–79.

Paulose-Ram, Ryne, Marc A. Safran, Bruce S. Jonas, Qiuping Gu, and Denise Orwig. "Trends in Psychotropic Medication Use among US Adults." *Pharmacoepidemiology and Drug Safety* 16, no. 5 (2007): 560–70.

Pearl, Betsy. "Ending the War on Drugs: By the Numbers." Center for American Progress, June 27, 2018. https://www.americanprogress.org/issues/criminal-justice/reports/2018/06/27/452819/ending-war-drugs-numbers/.

Penal Reform International. "Global Prison Trends 2021." Accessed November 28, 2021. https://www.penalreform.org/global-prison-trends-2021/.

Pescosolido, Bernice A., Jack K. Martin, J. Scott Long, Tait R. Medina, Jo C. Phelan, and Bruce G. Link. "'A Disease Like Any Other?': A Decade of Change in Public Reactions to Schizophrenia, Depression, and Alcohol Dependence." *American Journal of Psychiatry* 167, no. 11 (2010): 1321–30.

Petersen, Emily E., Nicole L. Davis, David Goodman, Shanna Cox, Nikki Mayes, Emily Johnston, Carla Syverson, et al. "Vital Signs: Pregnancy-Related Deaths, United States, 2011–2015, and Strategies for Prevention, 13 States, 2013–2017." *Morbidity and Mortality Weekly Report* 68, no. 18 (2019): 423–29.

Pew Charitable Trusts. "More Imprisonment Does Not Reduce State Drug Problems." Pew Charitable Trusts, March 8, 2018. https://www.pewtrusts.org/en/research-and-analysis/issue-briefs/2018/03/more-imprisonment-does-not-reduce-state-drug-problems.

Phelan, Jo C. "Geneticization of Deviant Behavior and Consequences for Stigma: The Case of Mental Illness." *Journal of Health and Social Behavior* 46, no. 4 (2005): 307–22.

Phelps, Michelle S. "The Paradox of Probation: Community Supervision in the Age of Mass Incarceration." *Law and Policy* 35, nos. 1–2 (2013): 51–80.

Pollack, Harold A., and Peter Reuter. "Does Tougher Enforcement Make Drugs More Expensive?" *Addiction* 109, no. 12 (2014): 1959–66.

Porter, Jane, and Hershel Jick. "Addiction Rare in Patients Treated with Narcotics." *New England Journal of Medicine* 302, no. 2 (1980): 123.

Prins, Seth J. "Does Transinstitutionalization Explain the Overrepresentation of People with Serious Mental Illnesses in the Criminal Justice System?" *Community Mental Health Journal* 47, no. 6 (2011): 716–22.

Prison Policy Initiative. "State and Federal Prison Wage Policies and Sourcing Information." Prison Policy Initiative, 2017. https://www.prisonpolicy.org/reports/wage_policies.html.

Provine, Doris Marie. "Race and Inequality in the War on Drugs." *Annual Review of Law and Social Science* 7, no. 1 (2011): 41–60. https://doi.org/10.1146/annurev-lawsocsci-102510-105445.

Provine, Doris Marie. *Unequal under the Law: Race in the War on Drugs.* Chicago: University of Chicago Press, 2007.

Puar, Jasbir K. *The Right to Maim: Debility, Capacity, Disability.* Durham, NC: Duke University Press, 2017.

Purdue Pharma. *OxyContin Marketing Plan, 2002.* Stamford, CT: Purdue Pharma, 2002.

Quinones, Sam. *Dreamland.* New York: Bloomsbury, 2016.

Ranapurwala, Shabbar I., Meghan E. Shanahan, Apostolos A. Alexandridis, Scott K. Proescholdbell, Rebecca B. Naumann, Daniel Edwards Jr., and Stephen W. Marshall. "Opioid Overdose Mortality among Former North Carolina Inmates: 2000–2015." *American Journal of Public Health* 108, no. 9 (2018): 1207–13.

Ray, Kristin N., Amalavoyal V. Chari, John Engberg, Marnie Bertolet, and Ateev Mehrotra. "Disparities in Time Spent Seeking Medical Care in the United States." *JAMA Internal Medicine* 175, no. 12 (2015): 1983–86.

Reedt, Louis, Kim Steven Hunt, James L. Parker, Melissa K. Reimer, and Kevin T. Maass. *Recidivism among Federal Drug Trafficking Offenders.* United States Sentencing Commission, 2017. https://www.ussc.gov/sites/default/files/pdf/research-and-publications/research-publications/2017/20170221_Recidivism-Drugs.pdf.

Reuter, Peter. "Why Has US Drug Policy Changed So Little over 30 Years?" *Crime and Justice* 42, no. 1 (2013): 75–140.

Rhee, Taeho Greg, and Robert A. Rosenheck. "Initiation of New Psychotropic Prescriptions without a Psychiatric Diagnosis among US Adults: Rates, Correlates, and National Trends from 2006 to 2015." *Health Services Research* 54, no. 1 (2019): 139–48.

Richie, Beth. *Compelled to Crime: The Gender Entrapment of Battered Black Women.* New York: Routledge, 1996.

Roberts, Dorothy. *Killing the Black Body: Race, Reproduction, and the Meaning of Liberty.* New York: Vintage, 2017.

Rose, Nikolas. "The Politics of Life Itself." *Theory, Culture, and Society* 18, no. 6 (2001): 1–30.

Rosenberger, Leif R. *America's Drug War Debacle.* Brookfield, VT: Ashgate, 1996.

Rothstein, Richard. *The Color of Law: A Forgotten History of How Our Government Segregated America.* New York: Liveright, 2017.

Sager, Alan. "Urban Hospital Closings: Why Care? What to Do? Policy and Financial Remedies for a Race-Linked Health Problem." Paper presented at the Annual Case Western Reserve University School of Law, Law-Medicine Symposium, 2014.

Sager, Alan, and Deborah Socolar. "Closing Hospitals in New York State Won't Save Money but Will Harm Access to Health Care." Boston: Boston University School of Public Health, 2006. https://www.bu.edu/sph/files/2015/05/Sager-Hospital-Closings-Short-Report-20Nov06.pdf.

Santo, Loredana, Pinyao Rui, and Jill J. Ashman. "Physician Office Visits at Which Benzodiazepines Were Prescribed: Findings from 2014–2016 National Ambulatory Medical Care Survey." *National Health Statistics Reports* 137 (January 2020): 1–16.

Sapolsky, Robert M. *Why Zebras Don't Get Ulcers: The Acclaimed Guide to Stress, Stress-Related Diseases, and Coping.* New York: Henry Holt, 2004.

Scher, Clara, Lauren Meador, Janet H. Van Cleave, and M. Carrington Reid. "Moving beyond Pain as the Fifth Vital Sign and Patient Satisfaction Scores to Improve Pain Care in the 21st Century." *Pain Management Nursing* 19, no. 2 (2018): 125–29.

Schmitt, Glenn R., Louis Reedt, and Kevin Blackwell. *Demographic Differences in Sentencing: An Update to the 2012 Booker Report.* United States Sentencing Commission, 2017. https://www.ussc.gov/sites/default/files/pdf/research-and-publications/research -publications/2017/20171114_Demographics.pdf.

Schnittker, Jason. "Social Distance in the Clinical Encounter: Interactional and Sociodemographic Foundations for Mistrust in Physicians." *Social Psychology Quarterly* 67, no. 3 (2004): 217–35.

Scott, Dylan. "16,932 People Have Lost Medicaid Coverage under Arkansas's Work Requirements." *Vox,* December 18, 2018. https://www.vox.com/policy-and-politics/2018 /12/18/18146261/arkansas-medicaid-work-requirements-enrollment.

Sentencing Project. "State-by-State Data." Washington, DC: Sentencing Project, 2020. https://www.sentencingproject.org/the-facts/.

Sentencing Project. "Trends in U.S. Corrections." Washington, DC: Sentencing Project, 2016. https://sentencingproject.org/wp-content/uploads/2016/01/Trends-in-US -Corrections.pdf.

Shelden, Randall G. *Controlling the Dangerous Classes: A Critical Introduction to the History of Criminal Justice.* Needham Heights, MA: Allyn and Bacon, 2001.

Shigematsu, Setsu. *Visions of Abolition: From Critical Resistance to a New Way of Life.* Riverside, CA: Visions of Abolition, 2012.

Sinclair, Elizabeth. *Going, Going, Gone: Trends and Consequences of Eliminating State Psychiatric Beds.* Arlington, VA: Treatment Advocacy Center, 2016.

Sinnenberg, Lauren E., Kathryn J. Wanner, Jeanmarie Perrone, Frances K. Barg, Karin V. Rhodes, and Zachary F. Meisel. "What Factors Affect Physicians' Decisions to Prescribe Opioids in Emergency Departments?" *MDM Policy and Practice* 2, no. 1 (2017): 1–8.

Smirnova, Michelle. "A Will to Youth: The Woman's Anti-aging Elixir." *Social Science and Medicine* 75, no. 7 (2012): 1236–43.

Smirnova, Michelle, and Jennifer Gatewood Owens. "Medicalized Addiction, Self-Medication, or Non-medical Prescription Drug Use? How Trust Figures into Incarcerated Women's Conceptualization of Illicit Prescription Drug Use." *Social Science and Medicine* 183 (April 2017): 106–15.

Smith, Brendan L. "Inappropriate Prescribing." *Monitor on Psychology* 43, no. 6 (2012): 36.

Smith, Sharon G., Xinjian Zhang, Kathleen C. Basile, Melissa T. Merrick, Jing Wang, Marcie-jo Kresnow, and Jieru Chen. *The National Intimate Partner and Sexual Violence Survey: 2015 Data Brief—Updated Release.* Washington, DC: Centers for Disease Control and Prevention, 2018.

Social Security. "SSI Federal Payment Amounts." 2022. Accessed September 7, 2020. https://www.ssa.gov/oact/cola/SSIamts.html.

Sommers, Benjamin D., Munira Z. Gunja, Kenneth Finegold, and Thomas Musco. "Changes in Self-Reported Insurance Coverage, Access to Care, and Health under the Affordable Care Act." *Journal of the American Medical Association* 314, no. 4 (2015): 366–74.

Springer, Gayle R. "Interrupting the School-to-Prison Pipeline: Are We Educating or Incarcerating Our Youth." Senior Honors Thesis, Eastern Michigan University, 2018. https://commons.emich.edu/honors/575.

Stafford, Randall S. "Regulating Off-Label Drug Use: Rethinking the Role of the FDA." *New England Journal of Medicine* 358, no. 14 (2008): 1427–29.

Steyee, Jimmy. *Program Performance Report: Implementation Grantees of the Adult Drug Court Discretionary Grant Program.* Rockville, MD: Bureau of Justice Assistance, 2013.

Stipek, Deborah, and Kathryn Hanson. "Schools vs Prisons: Education's the Way to Cut Prison Population." *San Jose Mercury News*, May 16, 2014. https://ed.stanford.edu/in-the-media/schools-v-prisons-educations-way-cut-prison-population-op-ed-deborah-stipek.

Strauss, Anselm, and Juliet Corbin. *Basics of Qualitative Research: Grounded Theory Procedures and Techniques.* 3rd ed. Thousand Oaks, CA: Sage, 1990.

Substance Abuse and Mental Health Services Administration. *Key Substance Use and Mental Health Indicators in the United States: Results from the 2018 National Survey on Drug Use and Health.* Rockville, MD: Center for Behavioral Health Statistics and Quality, 2019.

Substance Abuse and Mental Health Services Administration. *Key Substance Use and Mental Health Indicators in the United States: Results from the 2020 National Survey on Drug Use and Health.* Rockville, MD: Center for Behavioral Health Statistics and Quality, 2021.

Substance Abuse and Mental Health Services Administration. *Results from the 2013 National Survey on Drug Use and Health: Summary of National Findings.* Rockville, MD: Substance Abuse and Mental Health Services Administration, 2014.

Substance Abuse and Mental Health Services Administration. *Results from the 2014 National Survey on Drug Use and Health: Summary of National Findings.* Rockville, MD: Substance Abuse and Mental Health Services Administration, 2015.

Sue, Kimberly. *Getting Wrecked: Women, Incarceration, and the American Opioid Crisis.* Berkeley: University of California Press, 2019.

Szalavitz, Maia. *Unbroken Brain: A Revolutionary New Way of Understanding Addiction.* New York: St. Martin's, 2016.

Tamayo-Sarver, Joshua H., Susan W. Hinze, Rita K. Cydulka, and David W. Baker. "Racial and Ethnic Disparities in Emergency Department Analgesic Prescription." *American Journal of Public Health* 93, no. 12 (2003): 2067–73.

Tatum, Beverly Daniel. *Why Are All the Black Kids Sitting Together in the Cafeteria? And Other Conversations about Race.* New York: Basic Books, 2019.

Terry, Charles E. "Drug Addictions, a Public Health Problem." *American Journal of Public Health* 4, no. 1 (1914): 28–37.

Thielking, Megan. "Missouri Is the Only State Not Monitoring Prescription Drug Use. Will It Finally Create a Database?" *Stat News*, March 7, 2017. https://www.statnews .com/2017/03/07/missouri-prescription-drug-database/.

Thomas, Megan, and Cara James. *The Role of Health Coverage for Communities of Color.* Washington, DC: Kaiser Family Foundation, 2009.

Tiger, Rebecca. *Judging Addicts: Drug Courts and Coercion in the Justice System.* New York: New York University Press, 2012.

Tonmyr, Lil, and Margot Shields. "Childhood Sexual Abuse and Substance Abuse: A Gender Paradox?" *Child Abuse and Neglect* 63 (January 2017): 284–94.

Torrey, E. Fuller, Doris A. Fuller, Jeffery Geller, Carla Jacobs, and Kristina Ragosta. *No Room at the Inn: Trends and Consequences of Closing Public Psychiatric Hospitals.* Arlington, VA: Treatment Advocacy Center, 2012.

Torrey, E. Fuller, Aaron D. Kennard, Don Eslinger, Richard Lamb, and James Pavle. *More Mentally Ill Persons Are in Jails and Prisons than Hospitals: A Survey of the States.* Arlington, VA: Treatment Advocacy Center, 2010.

Torrey, E. Fuller, Mary T. Zdanowicz, Aaron D. Kennard, H. Richard Lamb, Donald F. Eslinger, Micheal I. Biasotti, and Doris A. Fuller. *The Treatment of Persons with Mental Illness in Prisons and Jails: A State Survey.* Arlington, VA: Treatment Advocacy Center, 2014.

"Undesirable Medical Advertisements Ordinance." Department of Health: The Government of the Hong Kong Special Administrative Region, 2022. https://www.drugoffice .gov.hk/eps/do/en/pharmaceutical_trade/other_useful_information/umao.html.

United Nations Development Programme. "Human Development Index." Human Development Reports, United Nations Development Programme, 2020. http://hdr.undp .org/en/composite/HDI.

United States Department of Education. "State and Local Expenditures on Corrections and Education." 2016. https://www.ed.gov/news/press-releases/report-increases -spending-corrections-far-outpace-education.

United States Department of Education, Office for Civil Rights. "2013–2014 Civil Rights Data Collection Data Snapshot: School Discipline." 2014. https://ocrdata.ed.gov/assets /downloads/CRDC-School-Discipline-Snapshot.pdf.

United States Department of Health and Human Services. *Sex, Race, and Ethnic Diversity of U.S. Health Occupations (2010–2012).* Health Resources and Services Administration. Rockville, MD: National Center for Health Workforce Analysis, 2015.

United States Department of Health and Human Services. "Who Is Eligible for Medicare?" 2014. https://www.hhs.gov/answers/medicare-and-medicaid/who-is-elibible-for -medicare/index.html.

United States Department of Justice. *Drug Enforcement Administration (DEA) History 1980–1985.* Washington, DC. Accessed March 30, 2022. https://www.dea.gov/sites /default/files/2021-04/1980-1985_p_49-58.pdf.

United States Department of Justice, Office of Justice Programs. "Bureau of Justice Statistics." 2022. http://www.ojp.usdoj.gov/bjs.

United States Food and Drug Administration. "FDA Drug Safety Communication: FDA Urges Caution about Withholding Opioid Addiction Medications from Patients Taking Benzodiazepines or CNS Depressants; Careful Medication Management

Can Reduce Risks." September 26, 2017. https://www.fda.gov/drugs/drug-safety-and
-availability/fda-drug-safety-communication-fda-urges-caution-about-withholding
-opioid-addiction-medications.

United States Sentencing Commission. *Mandatory Minimum Penalties for Drug Offense in the Federal Criminal Justice System*. Washington, DC: Government Printing Office, 2017.

United States Sentencing Commission. *2015 Report to the Congress: Impact of the Fair Sentencing Act of 2010*. 2015. https://www.ussc.gov/research/congressional-reports/2015
-report-congress-impact-fair-sentencing-act-2010.

Utsumi, Igor. "Advertising Regulation for Medication in Brazil." *Brazil Business*, January 17, 2015. https://thebrazilbusiness.com/article/advertising-regulation-for
-medication-in-brazil.

Van der Wees, Philip J., Alan M. Zaslavsky, and John Z. Ayanian. "Improvements in Health Status after Massachusetts Health Care Reform." *Milbank Quarterly* 91, no. 4 (2013): 663–89.

Van Ryn, Michelle, Diana Burgess, Jennifer Malat, and Joan Griffin. "Physicians' Perceptions of Patients' Social and Behavioral Characteristics and Race Disparities in Treatment Recommendations for Men with Coronary Artery Disease." *American Journal of Public Health* 96, no. 2 (2006): 351–57.

Van Ryn, Michelle, and Jane Burke. "The Effect of Patient Race and Socio-economic Status on Physicians' Perception of Patients." *Social Science and Medicine* 50, no. 6 (2000): 813–28.

Verona, Edelyn, Brett Murphy, and Shabnam Javdani. "Gendered Pathways: Violent Childhood Maltreatment, Sex Exchange, and Drug Use." *Psychology of Violence* 6, no. 1 (2016): 124–34.

Vila, Hector, Robert A. Smith, Michael J. Augustyniak, Peter A. Nagi, Roy G. Soto, Thomas W. Ross, Alan B. Cantor, Jennifer M. Strickland, and Rafael V. Miguel. "The Efficacy and Safety of Pain Management before and after Implementation of Hospital-Wide Pain Management Standards: Is Patient Safety Compromised by Treatment Based Solely on Numerical Pain Ratings?" *Anesthesia and Analgesia* 101, no. 2 (2005): 474–80.

Vrecko, Scott. "Birth of a Brain Disease: Science, the State and Addiction Neuropolitics." *History of the Human Sciences* 23, no. 4 (2010): 52–67.

Wacquant, Loïc. "Deadly Symbiosis: When Ghetto and Prison Meet and Mesh." *Punishment and Society* 3, no. 1 (2001): 95–133.

Wagner, Peter, and Wendy Sawyer. "Mass Incarceration: The Whole Pie 2018." Prison Policy Initiative, March 14, 2018. https://www.prisonpolicy.org/reports/pie2018.html.

Wailoo, Keith. *Pain: A Political History*. Baltimore, MD: Johns Hopkins University Press, 2014.

Wakeman, S. E., M. R. Larochelle, O. Ameli, C. E. Chaisson, J. T. McPheeters, and W. H. Crown. "Comparative Effectiveness of Different Treatment Pathways for Opioid Use Disorder." *JAMA Network Open* 3, no. 2 (2020): e1920622. https://doi.org/10.1001
/jamanetworkopen.2019.20622.

Wald, Johanna, and Daniel J. Losen. "Defining and Redirecting a School to Prison Pipeline." *New Directions for Youth Development*, no. 99 (2003): 9–15. https://doi.org/10
.1002/yd.51.

Walker, Renee E., Christopher R. Keane, and Jessica G. Burke. "Disparities and Access to Healthy Food in the United States: A Review of Food Deserts Literature." *Health and Place* 16, no. 5 (2010): 876–84.

Walters, Mikel, Jieru Chen, and Matthew Breiding. *National Intimate Partner and Sexual Violence Survey*. Atlanta, GA: National Center for Injury Prevention and Control, Centers for Disease Control and Prevention, 2013.

Wang, Jackie. *Carceral Capitalism: Building the Commune*. Cambridge, MA: MIT Press, 2018.

Warren, Carol A. B. "New Forms of Social Control: The Myth of Deinstitutionalization." *American Behavioral Scientist* 24, no. 6 (1981): 724–40.

Watkins-Hayes, Celeste. *Remaking a Life: How Women Living with HIV/AIDS Confront Inequality*. Berkeley: University of California Press, 2019.

Western, Bruce, and Becky Pettit. *Collateral Costs: Incarceration's Effect on Economic Mobility*. Washington, DC: Pew Charitable Trusts, 2010.

Western, Bruce, and Jake Rosenfeld. "Unions, Norms, and the Rise in US Wage Inequality." American Sociological Review 76, no. 4 (2011): 513–37.

Whiteis, David G. "Hospital and Community Characteristics in Closures of Urban Hospitals, 1980–87." *Public Health Report* 107, no. 4 (1992): 409–16.

Williams, Simon J., Paul Martin, and Jonathan Gabe. "The Pharmaceuticalisation of Society? A Framework for Analysis." *Sociology of Health and Illness* 33, no. 5 (2011): 710–25.

Wilson, Bobby M. *Golden Gulag: Prisons, Surplus, Crisis, and Opposition in Globalizing California*. American Crossroads. Berkeley: University of California Press, 2009.

Winchester, Mae-Lan, Parmida Shahiri, Emily Boevers-Solverson, Abigail Hartmann, Meghan Ross, Sharon Fitzgerald, and Marc Parrish. "Racial and Ethnic Differences in Urine Drug Screening on Labor and Delivery." *Maternal and Child Health Journal* 26 (January 2022): 124–30. https://doi.org/10.1007/s10995-021-03258-5.

Witt, Howard. "School Discipline Tougher on African Americans." *Chicago Tribune*, September 25, 2007. https://www.chicagotribune.com/chi-070924discipline-story.html.

Woolf, Steven H., Laudan Y. Aron, Lisa Dubay, Sarah M. Simon, Emily Zimmerman, and Kim Luk. *How Are Income and Wealth Linked to Health and Longevity?* Richmond: Virginia Commonwealth University, Center on Society and Health, 2016. https://www.urban.org/research/publication/how-are-income-and-wealth-linked-health-and-longevity/view/full_report.

Yearby, Ruqaiijah. "Racial Disparities in Health Status and Access to Healthcare: The Continuation of Inequality in the United States Due to Structural Racism." *American Journal of Economics and Sociology* 77, nos. 3–4 (2018): 1113–52.

Yeh, James S., Jessica M. Franklin, Jerry Avorn, Joan Landon, and Aaron S. Kesselheim. "Association of Industry Payments to Physicians with the Prescribing of Brand-Name Statins in Massachusetts." *JAMA Internal Medicine* 176, no. 6 (2016): 763–68.

Zgierska, Aleksandra, David Rabago, and Michael M. Miller. "Impact of Patient Satisfaction Ratings on Physicians and Clinical Care." *Patient Preference and Adherence* 8 (April 2014): 437–46.

Zola, Irving Kenneth. "Medicine as an Institution of Social Control." *Sociological Review* 20, no. 4 (1972): 487–504.

INDEX

Pastoral Clinic, The (Garcia), 88
patient-centered health care, 97–98
patient-prisoner, 42
patient satisfaction surveys, 28
Patrick (interviewee), 84–85, 88
Paul (interviewee), 57–58, 77
Penny (interviewee), 45–46
Percocet, 38, 49, 53, 60, 71, 79, 83, 86
pharmaceutical companies, 30, 34–35
pharmaceuticalization, 11–12, 18
pharmacists and pharmacies, 97
physician flight, 31
pleasure: as abuse, 7; as dysfunction, 69, 78; as
    illegitimate use, 19; and productivity, 8, 19;
    regulation of, 78
postpartum depression, 53, 55
poverty, 38, 107
pregnancy and childbirth, 51–53, 54
prescription drugs: data on, 27; getting hooked
    on, 47–58; proliferation of, 33–35; psycho-
    tropics, 2–3, 17–18, 22, 33–34, 80–82; as a
    technology, 11, 15; underprescribing, 64.
    See also specific drug names
prescription drug use: vs. abuse, 66, 68–70;
    legitimate and illegitimate, 66, 69, 78; licit
    and illicit, 7, 72–73; medical vs. nonmedical,
    4; moral aspects of, 40–41; normalization
    of, 3, 46–47; for pregnancy and childbirth,
    51–53, 54; racialized, 104–6; regulation of,
    7–8, 25, 71; for trauma, 55–58; for work,
    47–51. *See also* nonmedical use of prescrip-
    tion drugs; pain
prescription-to-prison pipeline, 15–19, 42–43,
    82–83, 90
preventive medicine, 30–31, 95–96, 102
primary care doctors, 3, 22, 31
prisons: *Are Prisons Obsolete*, 22; carceral
    continuum, 12–13, 103; mandatory minimum
    sentencing, 89–90, 100; mass incarcera-
    tion, 14; mental health care in, 80–82; net
    widening of, 92, 101; prescription-to-prison
    pipeline, 15–19, 42–43, 82–83, 90; prison
    abolitionist movement, 102, 103; school-to-
    prison pipeline, 16. *See also* criminalization;
    incarcerated people
probation, 101
productivity, 10
productivity and pleasure binary, 69, 78

professionals, privileging, 75–78
psychiatric institutions, 80
psychotherapy, 80, 97–98
psychotropics, 2–3, 17–18, 22, 33–34, 80–82
Puar, Jasbir K., 12
punitive model, reforming, 99–103
Purdue Pharma, 30, 35

Quaalude, 59
Quentin (interviewee), 86

race: Black incarceration rates, 22; colorblind
    racism, 21; health-care access and, 31–32;
    Negro dope fiend, 36, 38; overdose and, 15;
    prescription drug use and, 104–6; racialized
    addict, 35–40; and the War on Drugs, 14
Rachel (interviewee), 49–50, 83
rape, 55–58
Raphael (interviewee), 74–75
Rat Park project, 108
Reagan administration, 15, 90
recidivism, 101, 103
reforms: health-care, 95–99; in punishment,
    99–103; related to pain, 106–9; structural, 94
regulation of drugs, 102
rehabilitation programs: harm linked to, 6; im-
    pact of, 92; labels and, 69; patient-centered,
    97; as punishment, 100; significance of, 81;
    social problems in relation to, 13; surveil-
    lance in, 90–92. *See also* treatment
restorative justice, 103
Rhianna (interviewee), 47, 54
Richie, Beth, 84
Right to Maim, The (Puar), 12
risk factors, 48
Ritalin, 48, 58, 75
Ronald (interviewee), 47, 91

Sackler family, 34
SAMHSA (Substance Abuse and Mental Health
    Services Administration), 69
Sara (interviewee), 89
Schaaf, Rob, 89
school-to-prison pipeline, 16
sentencing disparities, 19
Seroquel, 58
Sessions, Jeff, 100–101
sexual abuse, 85

sexual violence, 55–58, 85
Shaun (interviewee), 63–65, 72
Silent Cells (Hatch), 81
slow death, as term, 9
sobriety, 91
social problems. *See* structural inequality;
    structural problems
social safety nets, 32–33
Sociologists for Women in Society, 113
Sonia (interviewee), 60
sports injuries, 63–64
Stacey (interviewee), 49, 74
storytelling, 109
structural inequality: identities and, 20–21;
    medicalization of, 11–13; and the opioid
    epidemic, 9–10; pain in relation to, 106;
    racialized aspects of, 65; racism and, 14.
    See also inequality; structural problems
structural problems: causes of, 25–26; genetic
    essentialism in relation to, 88; in health care,
    60; housing, 61; individual-level problems
    in relation to, 7; medicalization of, 24–25;
    as moral and biological problems, 18; phar-
    macological solutions for, 58–61; racism, 31;
    reforming, 94. *See also* structural inequality
Substance Abuse and Mental Health Services
    Administration (SAMHSA), 69
substance use vs. abuse, 25, 66, 68–70
Supplemental Security Income, 82
support and care, 97, 102–3, 107–9
surveillance and control: in the drug court sys-
    tem, 41–43; harm linked to, 6; in rehabilita-
    tion programs, 90–92; respectability linked
    to, 29; volume approach to, 90; of youth, 59

talk therapy, 61
therapeutic jurisprudence, 40–43
therapeutic turn, 8
tobacco, 39
Tonya (interviewee), 55
transformative justice, 103
transinstitutionalization and deinstitutional-
    ization, 81–83

trauma: childhood, 84–85; medicalization of,
    55–58, 106
treatment, 40–43, 59, 92, 97–98, 100, 101.
    See also rehabilitation programs
Trump administration, 100–101
Tylenol with codeine, 71

underprescribing, 64
unhoused people, 111–12
universal health care, 49

Valium, 35, 59
Vicodin, 2, 48, 49
Vietnam antiwar movement, 39
violence, sexual, 55–58
vital signs, 28
vulnerable populations, 111, 113

Wacquant, Loïc, 12–13
Wailoo, Keith, 30
waiver of documentation of consent, 113
Walter (interviewee), 50–51
Wang, Jackie, 103
War on Drugs, 7, 14, 15–16, 39–40, 102, 106
Watkins-Hayes, Celeste, 9, 104
white incarceration rates, 105
white middle-class mothers, 52
white prisoners, 14
white substance use, 104
white women and opium, 37
Whitney (interviewee), 57
withdrawal, 5, 18, 35, 45, 78, 98, 108
withholding medication, 98
work and prescription drugs, 47–51
World Health Organization (WHO), 7, 27,
    52–53

Xanax, 2, 57, 60, 64, 68

Yasmin (interviewee), 72

zero tolerance policies, 16
Zola, Irving K., 10–11

Printed and bound by CPI Group (UK) Ltd, Croydon, CR0 4YY

11/04/2023

03209751-0001